VEGETARIAN DIET FOR TWO

SPECIAL GUIDE AND COOKBOOKS FOR SINGLE PARENTS WITH KIDS WHO WANT TO FOLLOW A VEGETARIAN DIET TO IMPROVE HEALTH AND LOSE WEIGHT

(200 RECIPES)

TWO BOOKS IN ONE

By

Jim MOON

TABLE OF CONTENS

VEGETARIAN DIET GUIDE
HEALTH BENEFITS OF VEGETARIAN DIET

I've already mentioned some of the health benefits but let me back it up with some science. Of course, as mentioned earlier, if you eat only processed foods packed with sugar and saturated and trans-fat, eat little to no vegetables and fruits, and don't meet your macronutrient targets, you won't reap the benefits.

Boosts Heart Health

Following a plant-based diet makes you up to one-third less likely to end up in the hospital or die due to heart disease (Crowe et al., 2013). It all comes down to eating foods that will keep your blood sugar levels stable. High-fiber whole grains, nuts, legumes, and low-glycemic foods, in general, will reduce your overall risk of heart disease and lower your cholesterol (Harvard Medical School, 2020).

Reduces Cancer Risk

Vegetarians may have the upper hand when it comes to fighting off cancer (Tantamango-Bartley et al., 2013). This study found that plant-based diets don't only reduce your overall risk for cancer more than other diets; it is also more effective against female-specific cancers. Also, when it comes to Lacto- ovo vegetarians, they have a smaller chance of getting cancers of the gastrointestinal tract.

The consensus is that a diet filled with fresh fruits and veggies is key to combating cancer, and, of course, being a vegetarian makes it easier for you to get the recommended five servings a day.

Although the benefit isn't that significant, it is worth mentioning since every bit helps in the fight against the "big C."

Prevents Type 2 Diabetes

Following a healthy plant-based diet may prevent type 2 diabetes (Chiu et al., 2018). In fact, you have half the risk of developing this disease (Tonstad et al., 2013), and the good news doesn't stop there. If you already suffer from this disease, a vegetarian diet will help treat the associated symptoms and may even reverse the disease entirely (Jenkins et al., 2003).

Eating foods that keep your blood sugar levels steady is the secret behind preventing type 2 diabetes—something you'll be doing a lot of when you follow a vegetarian diet.

Lowers Blood Pressure

Plant foods are lower in fat and contain less sodium and cholesterol, which means they will help lower your blood pressure. Furthermore, fruits and veggies contain high potassium concentrations, which also help to lower blood pressure. Studies show that following a plant-based diet, primarily vegan, leads to lower blood pressure than those who consume animal products (Appleby et al., 2002).

Helps with Asthma

Animal foods trigger an allergy or inflammatory response in the body, so removing these foods from your diet will have a positive impact overall. One study (albeit an older one) found 22 out of 24 participants were less dependent on their asthma medication after adopting the vegetarian lifestyle (Lindahl et al., 1985).

Improves Your Mood

A lot of factors come into play when it comes to your mood—what you eat, how active you are, as well as your sleeping pattern. Since animal products are chemical-laden, cutting them from your diet will have a mood-boosting effect.

Increases Energy Levels Elevated energy levels are one of the most celebrated changes I noticed after switching to a vegetarian diet. There aren't enough hours in the day, but when you follow a plant-based diet, you have enough energy to do everything, and then some. Fruits and vegetables are high in vitamins and antioxidants, and this will give you a significant energy boost. The fact that your digestion will also run better due to the increased fiber will add to your newly-found get-up-and-go attitude!

Supports Better Sleep

Meat is heavy and can slow down digestion. When your body doesn't need to digest such dense proteins, you'll enjoy a better night's sleep. The speedier breakdown of plant protein also means your body will get all the minerals it needs for some much-needed shuteye. Add to that the fact that most vegetarians generally lead a healthier lifestyle—drink less, don't smoke, exercise regularly, etc., and counting sheep will be a thing of the past.

Improve Bone Health Osteoporosis is a leading cause of bone weakness, and this is caused by the removal of calcium from the bone and eventually leading to a hole in the bone. This condition is greatly reduced in people with a vegetarian diet. Eating animal products can lead to osteoporosis by forcing calcium out of the bone and eventually leading to less bone mineral. Those are some pretty amazing health benefits, right? And they're not the only ones—more and more studies are coming out documenting the positive bodily changes you'll experience if you cut out meat. Even a little goes a long way if you don't want to go full-blown vegetarian, try to steer your diet in a direction where the focus is more on fruits and veggies and less on meat. The Mediterranean diet comes to mind here!

WHAT TO EAT: MACRO- AND MICRO-NUTRIENTS

Since the standard American diet is built around animal protein, it's hard for most people to understand how vegetarians who reduce the ingredients they consider essential to a healthy diet will get the nutrients their bodies need. In fact, saturated fat and trans-fat in animal protein, antibiotics, chemicals, cholesterol, etc. are all harmful to the human body. If you learn about this, you will have to change your thinking about eating again In order to scientifically adjust your eating habits, I hope you have an understanding of protein, carbohydrates and fats, and understand how each nutrient is essential to the function of the body.

The best macronutrient breakdown for a vegetarian diet is as follows:

25% protein

45% carbohydrates

30% fat

If you're not sure what this means, you will need to work out how many calories your body needs per day to function at an optimal level. This depends on your body shape, age, activity level, etc. There are various calorie counters online that will help you calculate your daily caloric needs. Once you have this number, you just divide it in the above percentages, and "Bob's your uncle," as they say!

You will find people who will tell you that the vegetarian diet is too high in carbs. Well, not all carbs are the same Let me break down the various macronutrients and how much you need to eat to stay healthy. Afterward, we will look closer at the micronutrients.

Protein

Many vegetarians, both new and old, always have to deal with the problem of getting enough protein in their diet. The most important part of this is the confusion of how to deal with the choice of protein.

We both understand that protein is an essential part of a person's balanced diet. And most of our protein as humans comes from animals. But where will you get your protein from if you can't rely on a thick slice of steak? The truth is there are good numbers of protein sources from plants. As vegetarians, we have access to a wider variety of proteins, such as:

Tofu is the most familiar source of non-meat protein for a lot of vegetarians but believe me; there are many others I have tried and which you can too. Cooked Lentils; Cooked Beans; Whole Grain Pasta; Nuts; Eggplant; Tofu; Ground Flaxseed; Mushroom; Cauliflower; and Cooked Quinoa are some of the best sources of plant protein that you can add to maintain a balanced meal

It should now be clear that the belief that plant-based protein won't be enough to sustain your body's protein needs is unfounded. Ultimately, the building blocks of both types of protein (amino acids) are the same—on a cellular level, your body won't be able to tell the difference. Furthermore, when your body breaks down the amino acids in the food, it will build complete proteins. This also smashes the myth that you'll need to eat various proteins in one sitting to 'mimic' animal protein.

Carbohydrates

As I mentioned before, not all carbohydrates are created equal. Our body needs carbohydrates to function properly, but you must choose the right type of carbohydrates to get the best results. When choosing carbohydrates, the more natural the ingredients, the better for the body, because the simplicity of processing and packaging contains almost no fiber. However, foods rich in plant fiber, vitamins, minerals and phytonutrients can help your body resist oxidation and inflammation. Fiber content can slow down the digestion of carbohydrates and control the rise of blood sugar in the body. Eating high- fiber carbohydrates regularly helps you prevent type 2 diabetes, fight cancer, and keep your body in good condition.

As you read above, 45 percent of your daily calories should go to carbohydrates. If you follow a 2,000-calorie diet, you'll be eating 225 grams of carbs a day. However, you may end up eating more on a vegetarian diet, then you need to keep an eye on your carb intake to prevent weight gain.

Fat

I know you've been told that fat makes fat and leads to high cholesterol actually, people have misunderstood the role of fat for a long time. What's more, fat plays a vital role in your health. Fat is essential for the absorption of fat-soluble vitamins, cell growth, hormone production, and digestion. Research showed that eating good fats (polyunsaturated and monounsaturated) can help lose weight, reduce inflammation, fight depression and anxiety, and improve your overall health (Manikam, 2008).

Now that you know the importance of fat, I will tell you how to meet your daily fat needs from a vegetarian diet. First of all, it needs to be clear where we get good fats? Some foods include avocado (20 grams per 100 grams), soybeans (3.3 grams per cup), olives (3.2 grams per 28 grams) and pumpkin seeds (14 grams per tablespoon), both are good sources of fat. Another important thing is how to control the intake of fat in daily cooking.

☐Sauté food using water or vegetable broth. Make sure to check the liquid level frequently you don't want your food to burn. Just keep adding water or broth until your food is cooked. Fruit or vegetable purée and applesauce are great oil substitutes when you're baking. It will keep your cakes and other baked goods

moist.

☐If you're grilling something in the oven, I highly recommend getting a silicone mat to line your pan with. You can also use parchment paper to create the perfect non-stick environment for your oil-free grilling.

☐Invest in some non-stick cookware to help make cooking without oil less problematic. Okay, that covers your daily macronutrients. I think it's time we look at the vitamins and minerals (micronutrients) your body needs.

☐Vitamins and Minerals

As I mentioned before and will highlight throughout this cookbook, you need to focus on eating a wide variety of whole grains, fruits, vegetables, and fats with a particular focus on meeting your protein target if you want to get in all the nutrients your body needs. However, there are some nutrients you'll have to pay extra attention, or even consider supplementing.

Vitamin B-12

I want to take a moment to focus on vitamin B-12—a vital nutrient, which isn't found in many plant foods. If you decide to cut out all animal food sources, then you will have to consume more vitamin B-12-rich foods or you will have to supplement this vitamin. Since B-12 plays an important role in producing red blood cells and preventing anemia, I recommend you add a supplement to your diet just to be safe.

Omega-3 Fatty Acids

Before we move on to healthy foods you can't go wrong eating daily, let's look at omega-3s. To boost the health benefits of the vegetarian diet, getting in a good dose of fatty acids like docosahexaenoic acid (DHA), Eicosapentaenoic acid (EPA), and alpha-linolenic acid (ALA) is a must! Omega-3s help combat inflammation in the body, and through doing that, decrease your risk of getting heart disease or other issues caused by inflamed cells. When I first heard omega-3, I immediately thought about seafood, but I was pleasantly surprised that you could find ALA in various vegetarian sources.

HOW TO CHOOSE THE RIGHT FOOD FOR VEGETARIAN

Although all fruits and vegetables are superfoods as they're packed with nutrients our bodies love, some do stand out above the rest. Since making the healthiest choices is what you should aim for when following a vegetarian diet, you can boost your success rate by eating specific fruits and veggies daily, as well as focusing on herbs, spices, and drinks that have proven benefits.

I'll share with you some of the foods I attempt to eat daily and others I pack on my plate at least once a week.

Daily

Berries

Berries aren't only delicious, they're some of the healthiest foods on the planet. The number of health benefits packed in these juicy snacks is impressive. Not only do they contain essential nutrients, but they're also chock full of antioxidants that help keep free radicals at bay. What's a free radical, you ask? Well, they're rogue and unstable molecules that do you good in small numbers but will cause oxidative stress when their numbers get too high (LiveScience, 2016). This increases your risk of getting various diseases. But thanks to blueberries, blackberries, and raspberries and their high antioxidant content (the highest out of all common fruits), you can protect your cells (Wolfe et al., 2008).

Leafy greens

Kale, spinach, chard, and arugula are s78ome of the leafy-green superstars out there. They're low in calories but packed with vitamins, phytonutrients, and fiber. They're good for you in more ways than you can imagine. If the bulk of the veggies you eat is green and leafy, you can be sure to feel like a new person—even your skin will glow.

Nuts and seeds

Nuts and seeds are tiny yet powerful sources of protein, fat, fiber, vitamins, and minerals. What I appreciate most about these snacks is that I feel full and stay satiated for longer after eating only a handful. It's the perfect "tie-me- over" food when your tummy starts to grumble.

Turmeric

You've probably read about the wonders of turmeric or, more specifically, the active compound curcumin. This spice has scientifically been proven to have remarkable health benefits ranging from preventing heart disease, degenerative brain diseases, and can even help combat cancer cells. Its anti- inflammatory and antioxidant properties make it an anti-aging super spice.

Beans

If you ask me, one of the most underrated foods out there. Not only are beans and legumes high in dietary fiber, protein, vitamins, and minerals, they also contain B vitamins that you need as much of as you can get. Evidence suggests that beans' high fiber content will improve cholesterol levels and help your gut stay in good shape. Again, it comes down to managing those blood sugar levels!

Onions and garlic

You may not consider onions and garlic as nutritional powerhouses, but I am happy to convince you otherwise. Onions are high in potassium, folate, vitamin B6, and vitamin C. Garlic, on the other hand, contains all the goodies onions do with thiamin, calcium, phosphorus, copper, and manganese added to the mix!

And don't forget that it makes almost all savory dishes taste better.

Green tea

This wonder beverage is one of the healthiest on the planet. It comes loaded with antioxidants, which, as we've established, is terrific news for your overall health. Some of the health benefits of green tea include improved brain function, lowered risk of heart disease, protection against cancer, and better weight management (Chacko et al., 2010).

Once a Week

Ginger

Ginger is used in traditional and alternative medicine the world over, primarily when it comes to digestive health and fighting off nasty germs. Gingerol is the active compound in ginger and is responsible for all the medicinal properties. What makes it so powerful is the anti-inflammatory and antioxidant effects it has. You read about free radicals and oxidative stress and accompanied diseases earlier on, and now you have another food source to help heal your body!

Lemon juice

One of the main reasons why I can't do without lemon juice may surprise you. No, it's not for its vitamin C content but for its ability to combat anemia! Since vegetarians are prone to iron deficiency, including lemon juice in our diet will help with iron absorption from plant sources (Ballot et al., 1987). Your gut can absorb iron from animal protein, but it has a hard time doing so from plant-based sources. So, to help your body out a little, add lemon to your diet, as well as vitamin C and citric acid.

Dark chocolate

Who wouldn't want to eat chocolate once a week? I am not talking about overly sweet, processed, milk chocolate but the real deal—dark chocolate. The more unrefined the chocolate, the higher its flavanol content, and that's what we want. Flavanols are good for your arteries, and that makes them great for your heart and overall body. It tells your arteries to relax, and that reduces your blood pressure (Schewe et al., 2008). If you can recall, I suffered from hypertension when I first started following a vegetarian diet. Finding out that dark chocolate could help was delightful news!

Dates

This is another antioxidant-packed food, but that's not the only reason why I enjoy it once a week or so—dates make an excellent natural sweetener. Since they're dried, their sugar content is higher than fresh fruit, making them the perfect substitute for white sugar. Not to mention that they'll add some extra nutrients and fiber to any recipe you're preparing!

I usually make a date paste (recipe included in this cookbook) and substitute one cup of sugar with one cup of date paste.

However, you have to keep in mind that dried fruit overall has a much higher calorie content than their fresh counterparts. Furthermore, most of these calories come from carbs. That's my way of suggesting you don't overdo it when you eat this super sweet food—the vitamin, mineral, protein, and fiber content should blind you to the fact that it is a high-calorie food.

By now, you can understand my obsession too. I can be more serious once it comes to my vegetarian diet. In the pages that follow, there are mouth- watering recipes that will make you wonder why you didn't go meat-free ages ago. I also include some meal plans—something I found invaluable when I first started following the vegetarian diet. It makes it possible for you to stick to your guns and learn as you go along.

Note: This book has given you all the information you need to do this diet correctly and do it right. It is essential to understand what you are getting into when you embark on this diet, and this book gave you valuable information that you can use to your advantage and avoid the problems that can come with this diet. You want to stay healthy and make sure that your body can do what it needs to do. As with anything, we emphasize that if something seems wrong or unnatural, you will need to see a doctor to make sure you are safe and that your body can handle this diet. Use the knowledge in this book to get amazing recipes and learn directions for excellent meals for yourself. Consult your doctor before to starting new diet.

VEGETARIAN DIET FOR SINGLE PARENT
BREAKFAST RECIPES

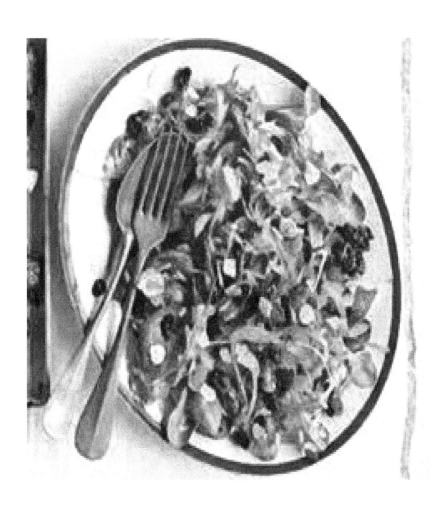

1) SPINACH SALAD

Preparation Time: 5 minutes   **Cooking Time:** 0 minutes   **Servings: 2**

Ingredients:

- ✓ 2 cups baby spinach
- ✓ 1 red bell pepper, roughly chopped
- ✓ 1 green bell pepper, roughly chopped
- ✓ ½ cup cherry tomatoes, halved
- ✓ 2 tablespoons olive oil

Ingredients:

- ✓ 1 teaspoon rosemary, dried
- ✓ 1 teaspoon basil, dried
- ✓ ½ teaspoon chili powder
- ✓ Salt and black pepper to the taste

Directions:

- ❖ In a bowl, combine the spinach with the peppers, tomatoes
- ❖ Add the other ingredients

- ❖ Toss and serve for breakfast.

2) ZUCCHINI BUTTER

Preparation Time: 10 minutes   **Cooking Time:** 0 minutes   **Servings: 6**

Ingredients:

- ✓ 3 tablespoons coconut oil, melted
- ✓ 1 pound zucchinis, grated
- ✓ 2 tablespoons coconut butter

Ingredients:

- ✓ A pinch of salt and black pepper
- ✓ 2 garlic cloves, minced
- ✓ 1 tablespoon chives, chopped
- ❖ Add butter and the other Ingredients

Directions:

- ❖ In a blender, combine the zucchinis with the coconut oil
- ❖ Pulse well. Divide into bowls and serve as a breakfast.

3) OREGANO PEPPERS BAKE

Preparation Time: 10 minutes   **Cooking Time:** 40 minutes   **Servings: 4**

Ingredients:

- ✓ ½ cup coconut milk
- ✓ 2 tablespoons flaxseed mixed with
- ✓ 3 tablespoons water
- ✓ Salt and black pepper to the taste
- ✓ 1 teaspoon oregano, dried
- ✓ 1 red bell pepper, cut into strips

Ingredients:

- ✓ 1 orange bell pepper, cut into strips
- ✓ 1 green bell pepper, cut into strips
- ✓ ½ cup chives, chopped
- ✓ 2 cups baby spinach
- ✓ Cooking spray

Directions:

- ❖ In a bowl, combine the peppers with the milk, flaxseed mix
- ❖ Then the other Ingredients except the cooking spray and stir.
- ❖ Grease a baking pan with the cooking spray

- ❖ Pour the peppers mix, spread and bake at 390 degrees F for 40 minutes.
- ❖ Divide the bake between plates and serve for breakfast.

4) ASPARAGUS AND AVOCADO BOWLS

Preparation Time: 5 minutes   **Cooking Time:** 6 minutes   **Servings: 4**

Ingredients:

- ✓ 1 tablespoon avocado oil
- ✓ 1 pound asparagus, trimmed and roughly sliced
- ✓ 2 avocados, peeled, pitted and sliced
- ✓ 2 tablespoons lemon juice

Ingredients:

- ✓ 1 tablespoon basil, chopped
- ✓ 2 teaspoons Dijon mustard
- ✓ 1 cup baby spinach
- ✓ Salt and black pepper to the taste

Directions:

- ❖ Heat up a pan with the oil over medium-high heat
- ❖ Add the asparagus, avocado, lemon juice and the other Ingredients

- ❖ Toss, cook for 6 minutes, divide into bowls and serve for breakfast

5) BERRY AND DATES OATMEAL

Preparation Time: 5 minutes **Cooking Time:** 0 minutes **Servings: 2**

Ingredients:

- ✓ ½ cup coconut flesh, unsweetened and shredded
- ✓ 1 cup coconut milk
- ✓ ¼ cup dates, chopped

Directions:

- ❖ In a bowl, combine the coconut flesh with the coconut milk

Ingredients:

- ✓ 1 teaspoon vanilla extract
- ✓ 1 tablespoon stevia
- ✓ 1 cup berries, mashed
- ❖ Add the dates and the other ingredients
- ❖ Whisk well, divide into 2 bowls and serve.

6) TOMATO OATMEAL

Preparation Time: 5 minutes **Cooking Time:** 20 minutes **Servings: 4**

Ingredients:

- ✓ 3 cups water
- ✓ 1 cup coconut milk
- ✓ 1 tablespoon avocado oil
- ✓ 1 cup coconut flesh, unsweetened and shredded

Directions:

- ❖ Meanwhile, heat up a pan with the oil over medium-high heat
- ❖ Add the tomatoes, chili powder and pepper flakes and sauté for 5 minutes
- ❖ Then the coconut and sauté for 5 minutes more.

Ingredients:

- ✓ ¼ cup cherry tomatoes, chopped
- ✓ A pinch of red pepper flakes
- ✓ 1 teaspoon chili powder
- ❖ Join also the remaining Ingredients, toss, bring to a simmer
- ❖ Cook over medium heat fro 10 minutes more
- ❖ Divide into bowls and serve for breakfast.

7) BREAKFAST BLUEBERRY MUFFINS

Preparation Time: 15 minutes **Cooking Time:** 25 minutes **Servings: 12**

Ingredients:

- ✓ Cooking spray
- ✓ 1 ½ cups rolled oats
- ✓ ¼ teaspoon baking soda
- ✓ 1 teaspoon baking powder
- ✓ ½ cup unsweetened applesauce
- ✓ ⅓ cup packed light brown sugar

Directions:

- ❖ Preheat your oven to 350 degrees F. Spray your muffin pan with oil.
- ❖ Add the oats in a food processor. Pulse until ground.
- ❖ Stir in the rest of the ingredients except blueberries. Pulse until smooth.

Ingredients:

- ✓ ¼ teaspoon salt
- ✓ 3 tablespoons vegetable oil
- ✓ 3 tablespoons water
- ✓ 1 tablespoon flax meal
- ✓ 1 teaspoon vanilla extract
- ✓ ¾ cup blueberries, sliced in half
- ❖ Pour the batter into the muffin pan. Top with the blueberries.
- ❖ Bake in the oven for 25 minutes. Store in a glass jar with lid.

8) OATMEAL WITH PEARS

Preparation Time: 15 minutes **Cooking Time:** 15 minutes **Servings: 1**

Ingredients:

- ✓ ¼ cup roll ed oats
- ✓ ¼ cup pear, sliced

Directions:

- ❖ Cook the oats according to the directions in the package.
- ❖ Stir in pear and ginger

Ingredients:

- ✓ 1/8 teaspoon ground ginger
- ✓ 1/8 teaspoon ground cinnamon
- ❖ Sprinkle with cinnamon
- ❖ Store in a glass jar with lid. Refrigerate overnight.

9) YOGURT WITH CUCUMBER

Preparation Time: 5 minutes   **Cooking Time:** 0 minute   **Servings: 1**

Ingredients:

- ✓ 1 cup soy yogurt
- ✓ ½ cucumber, diced
- ✓ ¼ teaspoon lemon zest

Directions:

- ❖ Put all the ingredients in a glass jar with lid

Ingredients:

- ✓ ¼ teaspoon freshly squeezed lemon juice
- ✓ Salt to taste
- ✓ Chopped mint leaves
- ❖ Refrigerate overnight or up to 2 days.

10) BREAKFAST CASSEROLE

Preparation Time: 20 minutes   **Cooking Time:** 43 minutes   **Servings: 6**

Ingredients:

- ✓ 10 oz. spinach
- ✓ 9 oz. artichoke hearts
- ✓ 2 cloves garlic, minced
- ✓ ¾ cup sun-dried tomatoes, chopped
- ✓ ½ teaspoon red pepper flakes

Directions:

- ❖ Squeeze the spinach to release the liquid. Add the spinach to a bowl.
- ❖ Stir in the artichoke hearts.
- ❖ In a pan over low heat, cook the garlic, tomatoes, red pepper
- ❖ Then lemon zest in oil for 3 minutes.
- ❖ Add the spinach and artichokes. Remove from heat.

Ingredients:

- ✓ 1 teaspoon lemon zest
- ✓ 1 tablespoon olive oil
- ✓ 2 cups almond milk
- ✓ 1 cup vegan cheese, crumbled
- ✓ 8 cups whole wheat bread, chopped
- ❖ Transfer to a baking pan.
- ❖ Stir in the spinach mixture and bread. Let sit for 30 minutes.
- ❖ Bake in the oven at 350 degrees F for 40 minutes
- ❖ Store in a food container and refrigerate.
- ❖ Reheat before serving.

11) COURGETTE RISOTTO

Preparation Time: 10 minutes   **Cooking Time:** 5 minutes   **Servings: 8**

Ingredients:

- ✓ 2 tablespoons olive oil
- ✓ 4 cloves garlic, finely chopped
- ✓ 1.5 pounds Arborio rice
- ✓ 6 tomatoes, chopped
- ✓ 2 teaspoons chopped rosemary
- ✓ 6 courgettes, finely diced

Directions:

- ❖ Place a large heavy bottomed pan over medium heat+ì
- ❖ Add oil. When the oil is heated, add onion and sauté until translucent.
- ❖ Stir in the tomatoes and cook until soft
- ❖ Next stir in the rice and rosemary. Mix well.

Ingredients:

- ✓ 1 ¼ cups peas, fresh or frozen
- ✓ 12 cups hot vegetable stock
- ✓ 1 cup chopped
- ✓ Salt to taste
- ✓ Freshly ground pepper
- ❖ Add half the stock and cook until dry
- ❖ Stir frequently. Add remaining stock and cook for 3-4 minutes.
- ❖ Then courgette and peas and cook until rice is tender
- ❖ Join also salt and pepper to taste.
- ❖ Stir in the basil. Let it sit for 5 minutes.

12) COUNTRY BREAKFAST CEREAL

Preparation Time: 5 minutes   **Cooking Time:** 40 minutes   **Servings: 6**

Ingredients:

- ✓ 1 cup brown rice, uncooked
- ✓ ½ cup raisins, seedless
- ✓ 1 tsp cinnamon, ground

Ingredients:

- ✓ ¼ Tbsp peanut butter
- ✓ 2 ¼ cups water Honey, to taste
- ✓ Nuts, toasted
- ❖ Simmer covered for 40 minutes until rice is tender

Directions:

- ❖ Combine rice, butter, raisins, and cinnamon in a saucepan
- ❖ Add 2 ¼ cups water. Bring to boil.
- ❖ Fluff with fork. Add honey and nuts to taste.

13) OATMEAL FRUIT SHAKE

Preparation Time: 10 minutes   **Cooking Time:** 0 minutes   **Servings: 2**

Ingredients:

- ✓ 1 cup oatmeal, already prepared, cooled
- ✓ 1 apple, cored, roughly chopped
- ✓ 1 banana, halved
- ✓ 1 cup baby spinach

Ingredients:

- ✓ 2 cups coconut water
- ✓ 2 cups ice, cubed
- ✓ ½ tsp ground cinnamon
- ✓ 1 tsp pure vanilla extract
- ❖ Blend from low to high for several minutes until smooth.

Directions:

- ❖ Add all ingredients to a blender.

14) AMARANTH BANANA BREAKFAST PORRIDGE

Preparation Time: 10 minutes   **Cooking Time:** 25 minutes   **Servings: 8**

Ingredients:

- ✓ 2 cup amaranth
- ✓ 2 cinnamon sticks
- ✓ 4 bananas, diced

Ingredients:

- ✓ 2 Tbsp chopped pecans
- ✓ 4 cups water

Directions:

- ❖ Combine the amaranth, water, and cinnamon sticks, and banana in a pot
- ❖ Cover and let simmer around 25 minutes.
- ❖ Remove from heat and discard the cinnamon. Places into bowls, and top with pecans.

15) GREEN GINGER SMOOTHIE

Preparation Time: 5 minutes   **Cooking Time:** 5 minutes   **Servings: 2**

Ingredients:

- ✓ 1 banana
- ✓ ½ apple sliced
- ✓ 1 orange sliced and peeled
- ✓ 1 lemon juice
- ✓ 2 big spinach

Ingredients:

- ✓ 1 tbsp. fresh ginger
- ✓ ½ cup almond milk
- ✓ For the dressing:
- ✓ Chia seeds, apple, raspberries

Directions:

- ❖ Take a blender. Peel off and slice all fruits
- ❖ Add banana, apple, orange, lime juice, ginger
- ❖ Then spinach and blend them well until they turn smooth
- ❖ Now add almond milk and pulse again for a few seconds
- ❖ Pour the smoothie into glasses and serve
- ❖ Add chia seeds, apple or raspberries for a smoothie bowl
- ❖ Store it up to 8-10 hours in the refrigerator.

16) ORANGE DREAM CREAMSICLE

Preparation Time: 5 minutes   **Cooking Time:** 5 minutes   **Servings: 2**

Ingredients:
- ✓ 1 orange, peeled
- ✓ ¼ cup vegan yogurt
- ✓ 2 tbsp. orange juice

Ingredients:
- ✓ ¼ tsp vanilla extract
- ✓ 4 ice cubes

Directions:
- ❖ In a blender, add orange, orange juice, vegan yogurt
- ❖ Then vanilla extract and ice cubes
- ❖ Blend all the ingredients well until smooth and well combined
- ❖ Pour it into smoothie glasses and serve.

17) STRAWBERRY LIMEADE

Preparation Time: 5 minutes   **Cooking Time:** 5 minutes   **Servings: 6**

Ingredients:
- ✓ 2 cup strawberries
- ✓ 1 cup sugar or as per taste
- ✓ 7 cups of water

Ingredients:
- ✓ 2 cup lemon juice
- ✓ Sliced berries for garnish

Directions:
- ❖ Take a small bowl, add sugar and water and put in microwave until dissolved.
- ❖ Now take a blender and add strawberries and a cup of water and blend well.
- ❖ Combine the strawberries puree with the sugar dissolve water and mix
- ❖ Pour lime juice and water if required
- ❖ Stir well and chill before serving
- ❖ You can add berries on the top as garnishing.

18) TOMATO AND ZUCCHINI FRITTERS

Preparation Time: 5 minutes   **Cooking Time:** 10 minutes   **Servings: 4**

Ingredients:
- ✓ 1 pound zucchinis, grated
- ✓ 2 tomatoes, cubed
- ✓ 2 garlic cloves, minced
- ✓ Salt and black pepper to the taste

Ingredients:
- ✓ 1 tablespoon coconut flour
- ✓ 1 tablespoon flaxseed mixed with 2 tablespoons water
- ✓ 1 tablespoon dill, chopped
- ✓ 2 tablespoons olive oil

Directions:
- ❖ In a bowl, mix the zucchinis with the tomatoes
- ❖ Add the other ingredients except the oil
- ❖ Stir well, shape medium fritters out of this mix and flatten them
- ❖ Heat up a pan with the oil over medium heat, add the fritters
- ❖ Cook them for 5 minutes on each side
- ❖ Divide between plates and serve for breakfast.

19) PEPPERS CASSEROLE

Preparation Time: 10 minutes   **Cooking Time:** 25 minutes   **Servings: 4**

Ingredients:

- ✓ 1 pound mixed bell peppers, cut into strips
- ✓ Salt and black pepper to the taste
- ✓ 4 scallions, chopped
- ✓ ½ teaspoon cumin, ground
- ✓ ½ teaspoon oregano, dried
- ✓ ½ teaspoon basil, dried

Directions:

- ❖ Heat up a pan with the oil over medium heat
- ❖ Add the scallions and the garlic and sauté for 5 minutes.
- ❖ Theb the rest of the ingredients except the cheese
- ❖ Stir and cook for 5 minutes more.

Ingredients:

- ✓ 2 garlic cloves, minced
- ✓ 1 tablespoon avocado oil
- ✓ 2 tomatoes, cubed
- ✓ 1.cup cashew cheese, grated
- ✓ 2.tablespoons parsley, chopped

- ❖ Sprinkle the cashew cheese on top
- ❖ Bake everything at 380 degrees F for 15 minutes.
- ❖ Divide the mix between plates and serve for breakfast.

20) LEEKS SPREAD

Preparation Time: 5 minutes   **Cooking Time:** 10 minutes   **Servings: 4**

Ingredients:

- ✓ 3 leeks, sliced
- ✓ 2 scallions, chopped
- ✓ 1 tablespoon avocado oil
- ✓ ¼ cup coconut cream

Directions:

- ❖ Heat up a pan with the oil over medium heat
- ❖ Add the scallions and the leeks and sauté for 5 minutes.
- ❖ Then the rest of the ingredients

Ingredients:

- ✓ Salt and black pepper to the taste
- ✓ ¼ teaspoon garlic powder
- ✓ ½ teaspoon thyme, dried
- ✓ 1 tablespoon cilantro, chopped
- ❖ Cook everything for 5 minutes more
- ❖ Blend using an immersion blender
- ❖ Divide into bowls and serve for breakfast.

LUNCH RECIPES

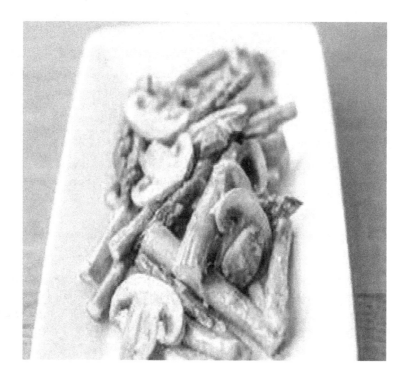

21) AVOCADO, ENDIVE AND ASPARAGUS MIX

Preparation Time: 10 minutes   **Cooking Time:** 10 minutes   **Servings: 4**

Ingredients:

- ✓ 3 avocados, peeled, pitted and sliced
- ✓ 2 endives, shredded
- ✓ 4 asparagus spears, trimmed and halved
- ✓ 2 tablespoons sesame seeds
- ✓ 2 tablespoons avocado oil

Ingredients:

- ✓ Juice of 1 lime
- ✓ A pinch of sea salt and black pepper
- ✓ Black pepper to the taste
- ✓ 1 tablespoon chives, chopped

Directions:

- ❖ Heat up a pan with the oil over medium heat
- ❖ Add the endives, asparagus, avocados and the other ingredients, toss
- ❖ Cook for 10 minutes, divide between plates and serve.

22) BELL PEPPERS AND SPINACH PAN

Preparation Time: 10 minutes   **Cooking Time:** 12 minutes   **Servings: 4**

Ingredients:

- ✓ 1 tablespoon olive oil
- ✓ 1 red bell pepper, cut into strips
- ✓ 1 green bell pepper, cut into strips
- ✓ 1 orange bell pepper, cut into strips
- ✓ 2 cups baby spinach

Ingredients:

- ✓ 3 garlic cloves, minced
- ✓ 2 teaspoons garlic powder
- ✓ A pinch of sea salt and black pepper
- ✓ 1 teaspoon fennel seeds, crushed
- ✓ 1 teaspoon chili powder

Directions:

- ❖ Heat up a pan with the oil over medium high heat
- ❖ Add the peppers and the garlic and sauté for 2 minutes.
- ❖ Then the spinach and the other Ingredients, toss
- ❖ Cook over medium heat for 10 minutes more
- ❖ Divide between plates and serve.

23) MUSHROOMS AND ASPARAGUS MIX

Preparation Time: 10 minutes   **Cooking Time:** 15 minutes   **Servings: 4**

Ingredients:

- ✓ 1 pound white mushrooms, sliced
- ✓ 1 asparagus bunch, trimmed and halved
- ✓ 1 teaspoon sweet paprika
- ✓ 1 teaspoon coriander, ground
- ✓ 1 teaspoon chili powder

Ingredients:

- ✓ ½ teaspoon thyme, dried
- ✓ 2 garlic cloves, minced
- ✓ ¼ cup coconut cream
- ✓ 1 tablespoon avocado oil

Directions:

- ❖ Heat up a pan with the oil over medium high heat
- ❖ Add the mushrooms, the asparagus and the other Ingredients, toss
- ❖ Cook for 15 minutes, divide between plates and serve.

24) KALE AND RAISINS

Preparation Time: 10 minutes   **Cooking Time:** 20 minutes   **Servings: 4**

Ingredients:

- ✓ 1 pound kale, torn
- ✓ 1 tomato, cubed
- ✓ 2 tablespoons avocado oil
- ✓ Juice of 1 lime
- ✓ ¼ cup raisins

Ingredients:

- ✓ 1 teaspoon nutmeg, ground
- ✓ ½ teaspoon ginger, grated
- ✓ ½ teaspoon cinnamon powder
- ✓ 1 tablespoon chives, chopped
- ✓ A pinch of sea salt and black pepper

Directions:

- ❖ Heat up a pan with the oil over medium heat
- ❖ Add the kale, tomato, lime juice and the other Ingredients, toss
- ❖ Cook for 20 minutes, divide into bowls and serve.

25) COLLARD GREENS AND GARLIC MIX

Preparation Time: 10 minutes   **Cooking Time:** 10 minutes   **Servings: 4**

Ingredients:

- ✓ 2 tablespoons avocado oil
- ✓ 4 garlic cloves, minced
- ✓ 4 bunches collard greens
- ✓ 1 tomato, cubed

Directions:

- ❖ Heat up a pan with the oil over medium heat
- ❖ Add the garlic, collard greens

Ingredients:

- ✓ A pinch of sea salt and black pepper
- ✓ Black pepper to the taste
- ✓ 1 tablespoon almonds, chopped

- ❖ Then the other ingredients, toss well
- ❖ Cook for 10 minutes, divide into bowls and serve.

26) CAULIFLOWER RICE AND CHIA MIX

Preparation Time: 10 minutes   **Cooking Time:** 15 minutes   **Servings: 4**

Ingredients:

- ✓ 2 cups cauliflower rice
- ✓ 2 tablespoons chia seeds
- ✓ ½ cup radishes, halved
- ✓ ½ cup chives, chopped

Directions:

- ❖ Heat up a pan with the oil over medium heat
- ❖ Add the cauliflower rice, chia seeds

Ingredients:

- ✓ 2 tablespoons avocado oil
- ✓ Zest of 1 lime, grated
- ✓ 1 cup coconut cream

- ❖ Add the other ingredients, toss
- ❖ Cook for 15 minutes, divide into bowls and serve.

27) FRUITY CAULIFLOWER RICE BOWLS

Preparation Time: 10 minutes   **Cooking Time:** 0 minutes   **Servings: 4**

Ingredients:

- ✓ ½ cup blackberries, halved
- ✓ ½ cup grapes, halved
- ✓ 2 cups cauliflower rice, steamed
- ✓ 1 cup cherry tomatoes, halved

Directions:

- ❖ In a salad bowl, combine the cauliflower rice with the berries

Ingredients:

- ✓ 1 avocado, peeled, pitted and cubed
- ✓ 2 tablespoons avocado oil
- ✓ Juice of 1 lime

- ❖ Add the other Ingredients, toss
- ❖ Divide into smaller bowls and serve.

28) SPICY ASIAN BROCCOLI

Preparation Time: 25 minutes   **Cooking Time:** 8 minutes   **Servings: 4**

Ingredients:

- ✓ 2 fresh limes' juice
- ✓ 2 small broccoli, cut into florets
- ✓ 2 teaspoon chili pepper, chopped

Directions:

- ❖ Add your broccoli florets into your steamer and steam them for 8 minutes.
- ❖ Meanwhile, to prepare dressing, add lime juice, garlic, chili pepper
- ❖ Then oil, and ginger in a small mixing bowl and combine

Ingredients:

- ✓ 2 tablespoons ginger, fresh, grated
- ✓ 4 garlic cloves, chopped
- ✓ 8 tablespoons olive oil

- ❖ Add steamed broccoli in a large mixing bowl
- ❖ Drizzle over it the dressing
- ❖ Toss to blend. Serve and enjoy!

29) TOMATO CUCUMBER CHEESE SALAD

Preparation Time: 15 minutes   **Cooking Time:** As per dierections   **Servings: 2**

Ingredients:

- ✓ 2 cups tomatoes, sliced
- ✓ 2 cucumbers, peeled, sliced
- ✓ 2 spring onions, sliced
- ✓ 7-ounces mozzarella cheese, chopped

Directions:

- ❖ In a large salad bowl, add basil pesto and cheese. Mix well

Ingredients:

- ✓ 12 black olives
- ✓ 2 teaspoons basil pesto
- ✓ 2 tablespoons extra-virgin olive oil
- ✓ 2 tablespoons basil, fresh, chopped
- ❖ Add remaining Ingredients into a bowl
- ❖ Toss to blend. Serve fresh and enjoy!

30) HEALTHY BRUSSELS SPROUT SALAD

Preparation Time: 15 minutes   **Cooking Time:** As per dierections   **Servings: 1**

Ingredients:

- ✓ ½ teaspoon apple cider vinegar
- ✓ 6 Brussels sprouts, washed, sliced
- ✓ 1 tablespoon Parmesan cheese, fresh, grated

Directions:

- ❖ Add all your Ingredients into a large salad bowl

Ingredients:

- ✓ 1 teaspoon extra-virgin olive oil
- ✓ ¼ teaspoon pepper
- ✓ ¼ teaspoon sea salt
- ❖ Toss to blend. Serve and enjoy!

31) HEALTHY BRAISED GARLIC KALE

Preparation Time: 50 minutes   **Cooking Time:** As directions   **Servings: 4**

Ingredients:

- ✓ 10 oz kale, stems removed and chopped
- ✓ 2 cups vegetable stock
- ✓ 4 tbsp coconut oil
- ✓ 1 tsp chili pepper flakes, dried

Directions:

- ❖ Heat coconut oil in a pan over medium heat.
- ❖ Once the oil is hot then add onion, garlic and chili pepper flakes
- ❖ Sauté until lightly brown. Pour vegetable stock and stir well.

Ingredients:

- ✓ 1 medium onion, sliced
- ✓ 4 garlic cloves, minced
- ✓ 1 tsp sea salt
- ❖ Now add chopped kale and season with salt. Stir well.
- ❖ Cover pan with lid and cook on low heat for 40 minutes.
- ❖ Serve and enjoy.

32) CAULIFLOWER LATKE

Preparation Time: 15 minutes   **Cooking Time:** 30 minutes   **Servings: 4**

Ingredients:

- ✓ 12 oz. cauliflower rice, cooked
- ✓ 1 egg, beaten
- ✓ 1/3 cup cornstarch

Directions:

- ❖ Squeeze excess water from the cauliflower rice using paper towels
- ❖ Place the cauliflower rice in a bowl.
- ❖ Stir in the egg and cornstarch
- ❖ Season with salt and pepper.
- ❖ Pour 2 tablespoons of oil into a pan over medium heat.

Ingredients:

- ✓ Salt and pepper to taste
- ✓ ¼ cup vegetable oil, divided
- ✓ Chopped onion chives
- ❖ Add 2 to 3 tablespoons of the cauliflower mixture into the pan
- ❖ Cook for 3 minutes per side or until golden.
- ❖ Repeat until you've used up the rest of the batter
- ❖ Garnish with chopped chives.

33) ROASTED BRUSSELS SPROUTS

Preparation Time: 30 minutes   **Cooking Time**: 20 minutes   **Servings: 4**

Ingredients:

- ✓ 1 lb. Brussels sprouts, sliced in half
- ✓ 1 shallot, chopped
- ✓ 1 tablespoon olive oil
- ✓ Salt and pepper to taste

Directions:

- ❖ Preheat your oven to 400 degrees F
- ❖ Coat the Brussels sprouts with oil.
- ❖ Sprinkle with salt and pepper.
- ❖ Transfer to a baking pan.

Ingredients:

- ✓ 2 teaspoons balsamic vinegar
- ✓ ¼ cup pomegranate seeds
- ✓ ¼ cup goat cheese, crumbled

- ❖ Roast in the oven for 20 minutes
- ❖ Drizzle with the vinegar.
- ❖ Sprinkle with the seeds and cheese before serving.

34) BRUSSELS SPROUTS & CRANBERRIES SALAD

Preparation Time: 10 minutes   **Cooking Time**: 0 minute   **Servings: 6**

Ingredients:

- ✓ 3 tablespoons lemon juice
- ✓ ¼ cup olive oil
- ✓ Salt and pepper to taste
- ✓ 1 lb. Brussels sprouts, sliced thinly

Directions:

- ❖ Mix the lemon juice, olive oil, salt and pepper in a bowl.

Ingredients:

- ✓ ¼ cup dried cranberries, chopped
- ✓ ½ cup pecans, toasted and chopped
- ✓ ½ cup vegan parmesan cheese, shaved

- ❖ Toss the Brussels sprouts, cranberries and pecans in this mixture
- ❖ Sprinkle the Parmesan cheese on top.

35) POTATO LATKE

Preparation Time: 15 minutes   **Cooking Time**: 10 minutes   **Servings: 6**

Ingredients:

- ✓ 3 eggs, beaten
- ✓ 1 onion, grated
- ✓ 1 ½ teaspoons baking powder
- ✓ Salt and pepper to taste

Directions:

- ❖ Preheat your oven to 400 degrees F.
- ❖ In a bowl, beat the eggs, onion, baking powder, salt and pepper
- ❖ Squeeze moisture from the shredded potatoes using paper towel
- ❖ Add potatoes to the egg mixture.

Ingredients:

- ✓ 2 lb. potatoes, peeled and grated
- ✓ ¼ cup all-purpose flour
- ✓ 4 tablespoons vegetable oil
- ✓ Chopped onion chives

- ❖ Stir in the flour. Pour the oil into a pan over medium heat.
- ❖ Cook a small amount of the batter for 3 to 4 minutes per side
- ❖ Repeat until the rest of the batter is used.
- ❖ Garnish with the chives.

36) BROCCOLI RABE

Preparation Time: 15 minutes   **Cooking Time:** 15 minutes   **Servings: 8**

Ingredients:

- ✓ 2.oranges, sliced in half
- ✓ 1 lb. broccoli rabe
- ✓ 1.tablespoons sesame oil, toasted

Directions:

- ❖ Pour the oil into a pan over medium heat
- ❖ Add the oranges and cook until caramelized
- ❖ Transfer to a plate.
- ❖ Put the broccoli in the pan
- ❖ Cook for 8 minutes

Ingredients:

- ✓ 1.Salt and pepper to taste
- ✓ 1 tablespoon sesame seeds, toasted

- ❖ Squeeze the oranges to release juice in a bowl.
- ❖ Stir in the oil, salt and pepper.
- ❖ Coat the broccoli rabe with the mixture
- ❖ Sprinkle seeds on top.

37) WHIPPED POTATOES

Preparation Time: 20 minutes   **Cooking Time:** 35 minutes   **Servings: 10**

Ingredients:

- ✓ 4 cups water
- ✓ 3 lb. potatoes, sliced into cubes
- ✓ 3 cloves garlic, crushed
- ✓ 6 tablespoons vegan butter
- ✓ 2 bay leaves

Directions:

- ❖ Boil the potatoes in water for 30 minutes or until tender. Drain.
- ❖ In a pan over medium heat, cook the garlic in butter for 1 minute
- ❖ Add the sage and cook for 5 more minutes.

Ingredients:

- ✓ 10 sage leaves
- ✓ ½ cup Vegan yogurt
- ✓ ¼ cup low-fat milk
- ✓ Salt to taste

- ❖ Discard the garlic. Use a fork to mash the potatoes.
- ❖ Whip using an electric mixer while gradually adding the butter, yogurt, and milk.
- ❖ Season with salt.

38) QUINOA AVOCADO SALAD

Preparation Time: 15 minutes   **Cooking Time:** 4 minutes   **Servings: 4**

Ingredients:

- ✓ 2 tablespoons balsamic vinegar
- ✓ ¼ cup cream
- ✓ ¼ cup buttermilk
- ✓ 5 tablespoons freshly squeezed lemon juice, divided
- ✓ 1 clove garlic, grated
- ✓ 2 tablespoons shallot, minced
- ✓ Salt and pepper to taste

Directions:

- ❖ Combine the vinegar, cream, milk, 1 tablespoon lemon juice
- ❖ Add garlic, shallot, salt and pepper in a bowl.
- ❖ Pour 1 tablespoon oil into a pan over medium heat
- ❖ Heat the quinoa for 4 minutes.
- ❖ Transfer quinoa to a plate.

Ingredients:

- ✓ 2 tablespoons avocado oil, divided
- ✓ 1 ¼ cups quinoa, cooked
- ✓ 2 heads endive, sliced
- ✓ 2 firm pears, sliced thinly
- ✓ 2 avocados, sliced
- ✓ ¼ cup fresh dill, chopped

- ❖ Toss the endive and pears in a mixture of remaining oil
- ❖ Add remaining lemon juice, salt and pepper.
- ❖ Transfer to a plate. Toss the avocado in the reserved dressing.
- ❖ Then to the plate. Top with the dill and quinoa.

39) ROASTED SWEET POTATOES

Preparation Time: 20 minutes **Cooking Time:** 20 minutes **Servings: 4**

Ingredients:

- ✓ 2 potatoes, sliced into wedges
- ✓ 2 tablespoons olive oil, divided
- ✓ Salt and pepper to taste
- ✓ 1 red bell pepper, chopped

Directions:

- ❖ Preheat your oven to 425 degrees F
- ❖ Toss the sweet potatoes in oil and salt
- ❖ Transfer to a baking pan.
- ❖ Roast for 20 minutes.
- ❖ In a bowl, combine the red bell pepper, cilantro, garlic and almonds

Ingredients:

- ✓ ¼ cup fresh cilantro, chopped
- ✓ 1 garlic, minced
- ✓ 2tablespoons almonds, toasted and sliced
- ✓ 1 tablespoon lime juice

- ❖ In another bowl, mix the lime juice, remaining oil, salt and pepper
- ❖ Drizzle this mixture over the red bell pepper mixture.
- ❖ Serve sweet potatoes with the red bell pepper mixture.

40) CAULIFLOWER SALAD

Preparation Time: 20 minutes **Cooking Time:** 15 minutes **Servings: 4**

Ingredients:

- ✓ 8 cups cauliflower florets
- ✓ 5 tablespoons olive oil, divided
- ✓ Salt and pepper to taste
- ✓ 1 cup parsley
- ✓ 1 clove garlic, minced

Directions:

- ❖ Preheat your oven to 425 degrees F.
- ❖ Toss the cauliflower in a mixture of 1 tablespoon olive oil, salt and pepper
- ❖ Place in a baking pan and roast for 15 minutes.

Ingredients:

- ✓ 2 tablespoons lemon juice
- ✓ ¼ cup almonds, toasted and sliced
- ✓ 3 cups arugula
- ✓ 2 tablespoons olives, sliced
- ✓ ¼ cup feta, crumbled

- ❖ Put the parsley, remaining oil, garlic, lemon juice, salt and pepper in a blender.
- ❖ Pulse until smooth
- ❖ Place the roasted cauliflower in a salad bowl.
- ❖ Stir in the rest of the ingredients along with the parsley dressing.

SNACK RECIPES

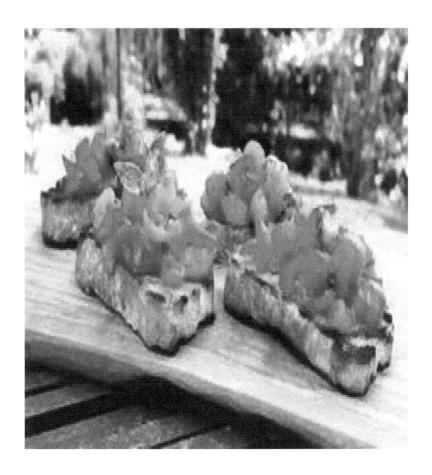

41) CANDIED ALMONDS

Preparation Time: 10 minutes   **Cooking Time:** 35minutes   **Servings: 4**

Ingredients:
- ✓ 1 cup sugar
- ✓ 1/2 cup water

Directions:
- ❖ In a pot over medium heat, boil water, cinnamon, and sugar
- ❖ Add almonds when water is boiling.
- ❖ Cook, stirring continuously, until liquid evaporates

Ingredients:
- ✓ 2 cups whole almonds
- ✓ 1 tbsp cinnamon

- ❖ Place almonds on a towel in a single layer to drain. Let cool 15 minutes.
- ❖ Serve.

42) STUFFED MUSHROOMS

Preparation Time: 10 minutes   **Cooking Time:** 20 minutes   **Servings: 12**

Ingredients:
- ✓ 1 tbsp vegetable oil
- ✓ 12 whole fresh mushrooms
- ✓ 1 tbsp minced garlic
- ✓ 1/4 cup grated Parmesan

Directions:
- ❖ Preheat oven to 350 degrees Fahrenheit and spray a baking sheet with nonstick cooking spray.
- ❖ Wash mushrooms, pat dry, and break off stems. Chop stems very finely.
- ❖ In a large skillet over medium heat, cook garlic and mushroom stems in oil until moisture evaporates
- ❖ Then remove from heat. Stir in cream cheese after cooling; add black pepper, Parmesan

Ingredients:
- ✓ 8oz packaged softened cream cheese
- ✓ 1/4 tsp onion powder
- ✓ 1/4 tsp black pepper
- ✓ 1/4 tsp ground cayenne pepper

- ❖ Join also onion powder, and cayenne pepper until thick.
- ❖ Fill each mushroom cap with mixture and place caps on baking sheet
- ❖ Bake for 20 minutes. Serve warm.

43) KETTLE CORN

Preparation Time: 5 minutes   **Cooking Time:** 10 minutes   **Servings: 5**

Ingredients:
- ✓ 1/2 cup unpopped popcorn kernels
- ✓ 1/4 cup white sugar

Directions:
- ❖ Heat oil in a pot over medium heat until hot but not smoking
- ❖ Stir in popcorn and sugar.
- ❖ Cover and shake constantly while popcorn is popping.

Ingredients:
- ✓ 1/4 cup vegetable oil

- ❖ When popping slows to 3 seconds between pops, remove from heat
- ❖ Continue shaking for 2 minutes more.
- ❖ Pour into a bowl and let cool. Serve.

44) BLOOMING ONION

Preparation Time: 10 minutes   **Cooking Time**: 10 minutes   **Servings: 4**

Ingredients:
- ✓ 1 cup milk
- ✓ 1 egg
- ✓ 1 cup flour
- ✓ 1-1/2 tsp cayenne pepper
- ✓ 1-1/2 tsp salt
- ✓ 1 tsp paprika

Directions:
- ❖ Beat egg and milk together in a large bowl.
- ❖ Combine salt, flour, cayenne pepper, black pepper, paprika
- ❖ Add thyme, oregano, and cumin in a separate bowl.
- ❖ Slice 1 inch from top and bottom of onion; peel off papery skin.
- ❖ Cut a 1 inch diameter core from the center of the onion with a thin knife.
- ❖ Slice 3/4 of the way through the onion with a sharp knife
- ❖ Then repeat in an X shape across the first slice. Continue until onion has been cut 12 to 16 times

Ingredients:
- ✓ 1/2 tsp black pepper
- ✓ 1/8 tsp thyme
- ✓ 1/3 tsp oregano
- ✓ 1/8 tsp cumin
- ✓ 3/4 cup vegetable oil
- ✓ 1 large onion

- ❖ Do this carefully so as to not break the onion all the way through
- ❖ Spread onion petals apart. Dip onion into egg mixture, then coat well with flour mixture
- ❖ Dip into egg mixture again, then coat with flour mixture again
- ❖ Heat oil to 350 degrees Fahrenheit in a fryer or deep pot.
- ❖ Fry right side up for 10 minutes or until brown, then remove and let drain before serving.

45) BRUSCHETTA

Preparation Time: 10 minutes   **Cooking Time**: 5 minutes   **Servings: 4**

Ingredients:
- ✓ 1/2 cup grated Romano cheese
- ✓ 5 tbsp mayonnaise
- ✓ 1/3 cup chopped red onion

Directions:
- ❖ Preheat oven broiler.
- ❖ Combine artichoke hearts with red onion, cheese, and mayonnaise in a large bowl,.

Ingredients:
- ✓ 6oz jar drained and chopped marinated artichoke hearts
- ✓ 1 French baguette, cut into 8 slices

- ❖ Spread equal amounts of mixture over bread slices. Place slices on a baking sheet.
- ❖ Broil for 2 minutes. Serve warm.

46) SPICY JALAPEÑO POPPERS

Preparation Time: 10 minutes   **Cooking Time**: 30 minutes   **Servings: 12**

Ingredients:
- ✓ 8oz shredded sharp cheddar cheese
- ✓ 8oz softened cream cheese
- ✓ 15 seeded jalapeño peppers halved lengthwise

Directions:
- ❖ Preheat oven to 350 degrees Fahrenheit; grease a baking sheet
- ❖ Combine cream cheese with mayonnaise and cheddar in a large bowl
- ❖ Stuff jalapeño halves with cheese mixture.

Ingredients:
- ✓ 1/4 cup mayonnaise
- ✓ 1/2 tbsp milk
- ✓ 2 beaten eggs
- ✓ 1-1/2 cups crushed corn flake cereal

- ❖ In a separate bowl, whisk eggs together with milk.
- ❖ Dip jalapeños into egg mixture, then roll in corn flakes to coat well
- ❖ Bake on baking sheet in a single layer for 30 minutes. Serve.

47) MEXICAN ROLL-UPS

Preparation Time: 10 minutes   **Cooking Time:** 0 minutes   **Servings: 8**

Ingredients:
- ✓ 8oz cream cheese
- ✓ 2/3 cup chopped green olives
- ✓ 1/3 cup mayonnaise
- ✓ 2 oz canned chopped black olives

Ingredients:
- ✓ 1/2 cup salsa
- ✓ 6 chopped green onions
- ✓ 8 flour tortillas

Directions:
- ❖ Combine cream cheese in a large bowl with green olives
- ❖ Add mayonnaise, black olives, and green onions.
- ❖ Thinly spread cream cheese mixture onto tortillas

- ❖ Roll up tightly and chill for 1 hour.
- ❖ Slice into pieces and serve topped with salsa.

48) BAKED ZUCCHINI

Preparation Time: 10 minutes   **Cooking Time:** 10 minutes   **Servings: 4**

Ingredients:
- ✓ 1/2 cup Italian bread crumbs
- ✓ 2 thinly sliced zucchinis
- ✓ 1/8 tsp black pepper

Ingredients:
- ✓ 2 tbsp grated Parmesan
- ✓ 2 egg whites

Directions:
- ❖ Preheat oven to 475 degrees Fahrenheit.
- ❖ Stir bread crumbs together with Parmesan and pepper in a small bowl
- ❖ Place egg whites in a separate small bowl.

- ❖ Dip zucchini slices into egg whites, then breadcrumb mixture
- ❖ Arrange in a single layer on a baking sheet.
- ❖ Bake for 5 minutes, flip, and bake for 5 more minutes. Serve.

49) PUMPKIN SEEDS

Preparation Time: 10 minutes   **Cooking Time:** 1hour   **Servings: 4**

Ingredients:
- ✓ 1/2 tsp salt
- ✓ 1-1/2 tbsp melted margarine
- ✓ 1/8 tsp garlic salt

Ingredients:
- ✓ 2 cups raw pumpkin seeds
- ✓ 2 tsp Worcestershire sauce

Directions:
- ❖ Preheat oven to 275 degrees Fahrenheit.
- ❖ In a large bowl, combine garlic salt, margarine, salt, and Worcestershire sauce.

- ❖ Stir pumpkin seeds into mixture. Place on a baking sheet.
- ❖ Bake for 1 hour, stirring a few times throughout. Let cool. Serve.

50) SPINACH BARS

Preparation Time: 10 minutes   **Cooking Time:** 40 minutes   **Servings: 12**

Ingredients:
- ✓ 1 cup flour
- ✓ 1 tsp baking powder
- ✓ 1 tsp salt
- ✓ 10oz rinsed and chopped fresh spinach
- ✓ 2 eggs

Ingredients:
- ✓ 1/2 cup melted butter
- ✓ 1 cup milk
- ✓ 1 chopped onion
- ✓ 8 oz shredded mozzarella cheese

Directions:
- ❖ Preheat oven to 375 degrees Fahrenheit and grease a baking dish.
- ❖ Boil spinach in a pot on the stove over medium-high heat
- ❖ When boiling, lower temperature to low
- ❖ Simmer for 3 minutes or until spinach is wilted. Drain spinach.

- ❖ Combine flour, baking powder, and salt in a large bowl
- ❖ Then stir in butter, eggs, milk, onion, spinach, and mozzarella.
- ❖ Place mixture in baking dish and spread evenly
- ❖ Bake for 35 minutes.
- ❖ Let cool, then slice into bars. Serve.

51) QUINOA BROCCOLI TOTS

Preparation Time: 10 minutes   **Cooking Time:** 20 minutes   **Servings: 16**

Ingredients:
- ✓ 2 tablespoons quinoa flour
- ✓ 2 cups steamed and chopped broccoli florets
- ✓ 1/2 cup nutritional yeast
- ✓ 1 teaspoon garlic powder

Ingredients:
- ✓ 1 teaspoon miso paste
- ✓ 2 flax eggs
- ✓ 2 tablespoons hummus

Directions:
- ❖ Place all the ingredients in a bowl, stir until well combined
- ❖ Then shape the mixture into sixteen small balls.
- ❖ Arrange the balls on a baking sheet lined with parchment paper

- ❖ Spray with oil and bake at 400 degrees F for 20 minutes until brown, turning halfway.
- ❖ When done, let the tots cool for 10 minutes.Serve straight away

52) SPICY ROASTED CHICKPEAS

Preparation Time: 10 minutes   **Cooking Time:** 20 minutes   **Servings: 6**

Ingredients:
- ✓ 30 ounces cooked chickpeas
- ✓ ½ teaspoon salt
- ✓ 2 teaspoons mustard powder

Ingredients:
- ✓ ½ teaspoon cayenne pepper
- ✓ 2 tablespoons olive oil

Directions:
- ❖ Place all the ingredients in a bowl and stir until well coated
- ❖ Then spread the chickpeas in an even layer on a baking sheet greased with oil.

- ❖ Bake the chickpeas for 20 minutes at 400 degrees F until golden brown and crispy
- ❖ Serve straight away.

53) NACHO KALE CHIPS

Preparation Time: 10 minutes   **Cooking Time:** 14 hours   **Servings: 10**

Ingredients:
- ✓ 2 bunches of curly kale
- ✓ 2 cups cashews, soaked, drained
- ✓ 1/2 cup chopped red bell pepper
- ✓ 1 teaspoon garlic powder
- ✓ 1 teaspoon salt
- ✓ 2 tablespoons red chili powder

Ingredients:
- ✓ 1/2 teaspoon smoked paprika
- ✓ 1/2 cup nutritional yeast
- ✓ 1 teaspoon cayenne
- ✓ 3 tablespoons lemon juice
- ✓ 3/4 cup water

Directions:
- ❖ Place all the ingredients except for kale in a food processor and pulse for 2 minutes until smooth.
- ❖ Place kale in a large bowl, pour in the blended mixture
- ❖ Mix until coated, and dehydrate for 14 hours at 120 degrees F until crispy.

- ❖ If dehydrator is not available, spread kale between two baking sheets
- ❖ Bake for 90 minutes at 225 degrees F until crispy, flipping halfway.
- ❖ When done, let chips cool for 15 minutes and then serve

54) RED SALSA

Preparation Time: 10 minutes   **Cooking Time:** 0 minute   **Servings: 8**

Ingredients:
- ✓ 30 ounces diced fire-roasted tomatoes
- ✓ 4 tablespoons diced green chilies
- ✓ 1 medium jalapeño pepper, deseeded
- ✓ 1/2 cup chopped green onion
- ✓ 1 cup chopped cilantro

Ingredients:
- ✓ 1 teaspoon minced garlic
- ✓ ½ teaspoon of sea salt
- ✓ 1 teaspoon ground cumin
- ✓ ¼ teaspoon stevia
- ✓ 3 tablespoons lime juice

Directions:
- ❖ Place all the ingredients in a food processor and process for 2 minutes until smooth.

- ❖ Tip the salsa in a bowl, taste to adjust seasoning and then serve.

55) TOMATO HUMMUS

Preparation Time: 5 minutes   **Cooking Time:** 0 minute   **Servings: 4**

Ingredients:
- ✓ 1/4 cup sun-dried tomatoes, without oil
- ✓ 1 ½ cups cooked chickpeas
- ✓ 1 teaspoon minced garlic
- ✓ 1/2 teaspoon salt

Ingredients:
- ✓ 2 tablespoons sesame oil
- ✓ 1 tablespoon lemon juice
- ✓ 1 tablespoon olive oil
- ✓ 1/4 cup of water

Directions:
- ❖ Place all the ingredients in a food processor
- ❖ Process for 2 minutes until smooth.

- ❖ Tip the hummus in a bowl
- ❖ Drizzle with more oil, and then serve straight away.

56) MARINATED MUSHROOMS

Preparation Time: 10 minutes   **Cooking Time:** 7 minutes   **Servings: 6**

Ingredients:
- ✓ 12 ounces small button mushrooms
- ✓ 1 teaspoon minced garlic
- ✓ 1/4 teaspoon dried thyme
- ✓ 1/2 teaspoon sea salt
- ✓ 1/2 teaspoon dried basil
- ✓ 1/2 teaspoon red pepper flakes

Ingredients:
- ✓ 1/4 teaspoon dried oregano
- ✓ 1/2 teaspoon maple syrup
- ✓ 1/4 cup apple cider vinegar
- ✓ 1/4 cup and 1 teaspoon olive oil
- ✓ 2 tablespoons chopped parsley

Directions:
- ❖ Take a skillet pan, place it over medium-high heat
- ❖ Add 1 teaspoon oil and when hot, add mushrooms
- ❖ Cook for 5 minutes until golden brown.

- ❖ Meanwhile, prepare the marinade and for this, place remaining ingredients in a bowl
- ❖ Whisk until combined. When mushrooms have cooked, transfer them into the bowl of marinade
- ❖ Toss until well coated. Serve straight away

57) HUMMUS QUESADILLAS

Preparation Time: 5 minutes   **Cooking Time:** 15 minutes   **Servings: 1**

Ingredients:
- ✓ 1 tortilla, whole wheat
- ✓ 1/4 cup diced roasted red peppers
- ✓ 1 cup baby spinach
- ✓ 1/3 teaspoon minced garlic
- ✓ ¼ teaspoon salt

Ingredients:
- ✓ ¼ teaspoon ground black pepper
- ✓ 1/4 teaspoon olive oil
- ✓ 1/4 cup hummus
- ✓ Oil as needed

Directions:
- ❖ Place a large pan over medium heat
- ❖ Add oil and when hot, add red peppers and garlic
- ❖ Season with salt and black pepper and cook for 3 minutes until sauté.
- ❖ Then stir in spinach, cook for 1 minute
- ❖ Remove the pan from heat and transfer the mixture in a bowl.

- ❖ Prepare quesadilla and for this, spread hummus on one-half of the tortilla
- ❖ Then spread spinach mixture on it, cover the filling with the other half of the tortilla
- ❖ Cook in a pan for 3 minutes per side until browned.
- ❖ When done, cut the quesadilla into wedges and serve

58) NACHO CHEESE SAUCE

Preparation Time: 5 minutes   **Cooking Time:** 10 minutes   **Servings: 4**

Ingredients:
- ✓ 3 tablespoons flour
- ✓ 1/4 teaspoon garlic salt
- ✓ 1/4 teaspoon salt
- ✓ 1/2 teaspoon cumin
- ✓ 1/4 teaspoon paprika

Ingredients:
- ✓ 1 teaspoon red chili powder
- ✓ 1/8 teaspoon cayenne powder
- ✓ 1 cup vegan cashew yogurt
- ✓ 1 1/4 cups vegetable broth

Directions:
- ❖ Take a small saucepan, place it over medium heat
- ❖ Pour in vegetable broth, and bring it to a boil.
- ❖ Then whisk together flour and yogurt, add to the boiling broth

- ❖ Stir in all the spices, switch heat to medium-low level
- ❖ Cook for 5 minutes until thickened. Serve straight away.

59) AVOCADO TOMATO BRUSCHETTA

Preparation Time: 10 minutes   **Cooking Time:** 0 minute   **Servings: 4**

Ingredients:
- ✓ 3 slices of whole-grain bread
- ✓ 6 chopped cherry tomatoes
- ✓ ½ of sliced avocado
- ✓ ½ teaspoon minced garlic

Ingredients:
- ✓ ½ teaspoon ground black pepper
- ✓ 2 tablespoons chopped basil
- ✓ ½ teaspoon of sea salt
- ✓ 1 teaspoon balsamic vinegar

Directions:
- ❖ Place tomatoes in a bowl, and then stir in vinegar until mixed.
- ❖ Top bread slices with avocado slices

- ❖ Then top evenly with tomato mixture, garlic and basil
- ❖ Season with salt and black pepper. Serve straight away

60) CINNAMON BANANAS

Preparation Time: 5 minutes   **Cooking Time:** 8 minutes   **Servings: 2**

Ingredients:
- ✓ 2 bananas, peeled, sliced
- ✓ 1 teaspoon cinnamon

Ingredients:
- ✓ 2 tablespoons granulated Splenda
- ✓ 1/4 teaspoon nutmeg

Directions:
- ❖ Prepare the cinnamon mixture and for this, place all the ingredients in a bowl, except for banana
- ❖ Stir until mixed. Take a large skillet pan, place it over medium heat
- ❖ Spray with oil, add banana slices and sprinkle with half of the prepared cinnamon mixture.

- ❖ Cook for 3 minutes, then sprinkle with remaining prepared cinnamon mixture
- ❖ Continue to cook for 3 minutes until tender and hot. Serve straight away

DINNER RECIPES

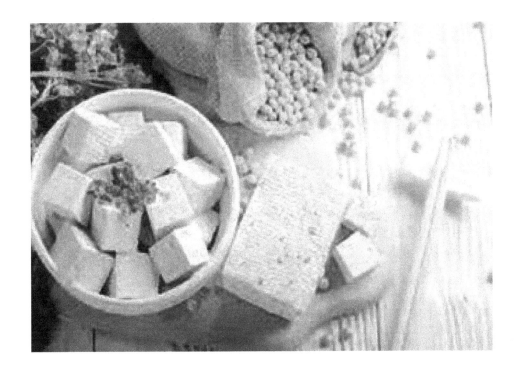

61) GINGER LIME TEMPEH

Preparation Time: 10 minutes   **Cooking Time:** 40 minutes   **Servings: 4**

Ingredients:
- ✓ 5 kaffir lime leaves
- ✓ 1 tbsp cumin powder
- ✓ 1 tbsp ginger powder
- ✓ 1 cup plain unsweetened yogurt

Directions:

- ❖ In a large bowl, combine the kaffir lime leaves, cumin, ginger, and plain yogurt
- ❖ Add the tempeh, season with salt, and black pepper, and mix to coat well
- ❖ Cover the bowl with a plastic wrap and marinate in the refrigerator for 2 to 3 hours.
- ❖ Preheat the oven to 350 f and grease a baking sheet with cooking spray.
- ❖ Take out the tempeh and arrange on the baking sheet

Ingredients:
- ✓ 2 lb tempeh
- ✓ Salt and ground black pepper to taste
- ✓ 1 tbsp olive oil
- ✓ 1 limes, juiced

- ❖ Drizzle with olive oil, lime juice, cover with aluminum foil
- ❖ Slow-cook in the oven for 1 to 1 ½ hours or until the tempeh cooks within.
- ❖ Remove the aluminum foil, turn the broiler side of the oven on
- ❖ Brown the top of the tempeh for 5 to 10 minutes.
- ❖ Take out the tempeh and serve warm with red cabbage slaw.

62) TOFU MOZZARELLA

Preparation Time: 10minutes   **Cooking Time:** 35minutes   **Servings: 4**

Ingredients:
- ✓ 1½ lb tofu, halved lengthwise
- ✓ Salt and ground black pepper to taste
- ✓ 2 eggs
- ✓ 2 tbsp italian seasoning
- ✓ 1 pinch red chili flakes
- ✓ ½ cup sliced pecorino romano cheese
- ✓ ¼ cup fresh parsley, chopped

Directions:

- ❖ Preheat the oven to 400 f and grease a baking dish with cooking spray. Set aside.
- ❖ Season the tofu with salt and black pepper; set aside.
- ❖ In a medium bowl, whisk the eggs with the italian seasoning, and red chili flakes
- ❖ In a plate, combine the pecorino romano cheese with parsley.
- ❖ Melt the butter in a medium skillet over medium heat.
- ❖ Quickly dip the tofu in the egg mixture and then dredge generously in the cheese mixture
- ❖ Place in the butter and fry on both sides
- ❖ (Until the cheese melts and is golden brown, 8 to 10 minutes)

Ingredients:
- ✓ 4 tbsp butter
- ✓ 2 garlic cloves, minced
- ✓ 2 cups crushed tomatoes
- ✓ 1 tbsp dried basil
- ✓ Salt and ground black pepper to taste
- ✓ ½ lb sliced mozzarella cheese

- ❖ Place on a plate and set aside.
- ❖ Sauté the garlic in the same pan and mix in the tomatoes
- ❖ Top with the basil, salt, and black pepper
- ❖ Cook for 5 to 10 minutes. Pour the sauce into the baking dish.
- ❖ Lay the tofu pieces in the sauce and top with the mozzarella cheese
- ❖ Bake in the oven for 10 to 15 minutes or until the cheese melts completely.
- ❖ Remove the dish and serve with leafy green salad.

63) SEITAN MEATZA WITH KALE

Preparation Time: 10minutes   **Cooking Time:** 22minutes   **Servings: 4**

Ingredients:
- ✓ 1 lb ground seitan
- ✓ Salt and black pepper to taste
- ✓ 2 cups powdered parmesan cheese
- ✓ ¼ tsp onion powder
- ✓ ¼ tsp garlic powder

Ingredients:
- ✓ ½ cup unsweetened tomato sauce
- ✓ 1 tsp white vinegar
- ✓ ½ tsp liquid smoke
- ✓ ¼ cup baby kale, chopped roughly
- ✓ 1 cup mozzarella cheese

Directions:
- ❖ Preheat the oven to 400 f and line a medium pizza pan with parchment paper
- ❖ Grease with cooking spray. Set aside.
- ❖ In a medium bowl, combine the seitan, salt, black pepper, and parmesan cheese
- ❖ Spread the mixture on the pizza pan to fit the shape of the pan
- ❖ Bake in the oven for 15 minutes or until the meat cooks.

- ❖ Meanwhile in a medium bowl, mix the onion powder, garlic powder
- ❖ Add tomato sauce, vinegar, and liquid smoke.
- ❖ Remove the meat crust from the oven and spread the tomato mixture on top
- ❖ Add the kale and sprinkle with the mozzarella cheese.
- ❖ Bake in the oven for 7 minutes or until the cheese melts.
- ❖ Take out from the oven, slice, and serve warm.

64) TACO TEMPEH CASSEROLE

Preparation Time: 10minutes   **Cooking Time:** 20minutes   **Servings: 4**

Ingredients:
- ✓ 1 tempeh, shredded
- ✓ 1/3 cup vegan mayonnaise
- ✓ 8 oz dairy- free cream cheese (vegan 1 yellow onion, sliced
- ✓ 1 yellow bell pepper, deseeded and chopped

Ingredients:
- ✓ 2 tbsp taco seasoning
- ✓ ½ cup shredded cheddar cheese
- ✓ Salt and ground black pepper to taste

Directions:
- ❖ Preheat the oven to 400 f and grease a baking dish with cooking spray.
- ❖ Into the dish, put the tempeh, mayonnaise, cashew cream, onion
- ❖ Then bell pepper, taco seasoning, and two-thirds of the cheese, salt, and black pepper

- ❖ Mix the ingredients and top with the remaining cheese.
- ❖ Bake in the oven for 15 to 20 minutes or until the cheese melts and is golden brown.
- ❖ Remove the dish, plate, and serve with lettuce leaves

65) BROCCOLI TEMPEH ALFREDO

Preparation Time: 10minutes   **Cooking Time:** 15minutes   **Servings: 4**

Ingredients:
- ✓ 6 slices tempeh, chopped
- ✓ 2 tbsp butter
- ✓ 4 tofu, cut into 1-inch cubes
- ✓ Salt and ground black pepper to taste
- ✓ 4 garlic cloves, minced

Directions:
- ❖ Put the tempeh in a medium skillet over medium heat and fry until crispy and brown, 5 minutes.
- ❖ Spoon onto a plate and set aside. Melt the butter in the same skillet
- ❖ Season the tofu with salt and black pepper, and cook on both sides until goldern brown
- ❖ Spoon onto the tempeh's plate and set aside.
- ❖ Add the garlic to the skillet, sauté for 1 minute.
- ❖ Mix in the full- fat heavy cream, tofu, and tempeh, and kale
- ❖ Allow simmering for 5 minutes or until the sauce thickens.

Ingredients:
- ✓ 1 cup baby kale, chopped
- ✓ 1 ½ cups full- fat heavy cream
- ✓ 1 medium head broccoli, cut into florets
- ✓ ¼ cup shredded parmesan cheese directions:

- ❖ Meanwhile, pour the broccoli into a large safe-microwave bowl
- ❖ Sprinkle with some water, season with salt, and black pepper
- ❖ Microwave for 2 minutes or until the broccoli softens.
- ❖ Spoon the broccoli into the sauce, top with the parmesan cheese
- ❖ Stir and cook until the cheese melts. Turn the heat off.
- ❖ Spoon the mixture into a serving platter and serve warm

66) AVOCADO SEITAN

Preparation Time: 10 minutes   **Cooking Time:** 2 hours 15 minutes   **Servings: 4**

Ingredients:
- ✓ 1 white onion, finely chopped
- ✓ ¼ cup vegetable stock
- ✓ 3 tbsp coconut oil
- ✓ 3 tbsp tamari sauce
- ✓ 3 tbsp chili pepper

Directions:
- ❖ In a large pot, combine the onion, vegetable stock, coconut oil
- ❖ Then tamari sauce, chili pepper, red wine vinegar, salt, black pepper
- ❖ Add the seitan, close the lid, and cook over low heat for 2 hours.

Ingredients:
- ✓ 1 tbsp red wine vinegar
- ✓ Salt and ground black pepper to taste
- ✓ 2 lb seitan
- ✓ 1 large avocado, halved and pitted
- ✓ ½ lemon, juiced

- ❖ Scoop the avocado pulp into a bowl, add the lemon juice, and using a fork
- ❖ Mash the avocado into a puree. Set aside.
- ❖ When ready, turn the heat off and mix in the avocado
- ❖ Adjust the taste with salt and black pepper.
- ❖ Spoon onto a serving platter and serve warm

67) SEITAN MUSHROOM BURGERS

Preparation Time: 15 minutes   **Cooking Time:** 13 minutes   **Servings: 4**

Ingredients:
- ✓ 1 ½ lb ground seitan
- ✓ Salt and ground black pepper to taste 1 tbsp unsweetened tomato sauce
- ✓ 6 large portobello caps, destemmed 1 tbsp olive oil
- ✓ 6 slices cheddar cheese for topping:

Ingredients:
- ✓ 4 lettuce leaves
- ✓ 4 large tomato slices
- ✓ ¼ cup mayonnaise

Directions:
- ❖ In a medium bowl, combine the seitan, salt, black pepper, and tomato sauce
- ❖ Use your hands, mold the mixture into 4 patties, and set aside.
- ❖ Rinse the mushrooms under running water and pat dry.
- ❖ Heat the olive oil in a medium skillet
- ❖ Place in the portobello caps and cook until softened, 3 to 4 minutes
- ❖ Transfer to a serving plate and set aside.

- ❖ Put the seitan patties in the skillet and fry on both sides (
- ❖ Until brown and compacted, 8 minutes)
- ❖ Place the vegan cheddar slices on the food
- ❖ Allow melting for 1 minute and lift each patty onto each mushroom cap.
- ❖ Divide the lettuce on top, then the tomato slices,
- ❖ Add some mayonnaise. Serve immediately.

68) TACO TEMPEH STUFFED PEPPERS

Preparation Time: 15 minutes   **Cooking Time:** 41 minutes   **Servings: 6**

Ingredients:
- ✓ 6 yellow bell peppers, halved and deseeded
- ✓ 1 ½ tbsp olive oil
- ✓ Salt and ground black pepper to taste
- ✓ 3 tbsp butter
- ✓ 3 garlic cloves, minced

Ingredients:
- ✓ ½ white onion, chopped
- ✓ 2 lbs. Ground tempeh
- ✓ 3 tsp taco seasoning
- ✓ 1 cup riced broccoli
- ✓ ¼ cup grated cheddar cheese
- ✓ Plain unsweetened yogurt for serving

Directions:
- ❖ Preheat the oven to 400 f and grease a baking dish with cooking spray. Set aside.
- ❖ Drizzle the bell peppers with the olive oil and season with some salt. Set aside.
- ❖ Melt the butter in a large skillet and sauté the garlic and onion for 3 minutes
- ❖ Stir in the tempeh, taco seasoning, salt, and black pepper
- ❖ Cook until the meat is no longer pink, 8 minutes.
- ❖ Mix in the broccoli until adequately incorporated. Turn the heat off.

- ❖ Spoon the mixture into the peppers, top with the cheddar cheese
- ❖ Place the peppers in the baking dish
- ❖ Bake in the oven until the cheese melts and is bubbly, 30 minutes.
- ❖ Remove the dish from the oven and plate the peppers
- ❖ Top with the palin yogurt and serve warm.

69) TANGY TOFU MEATLOAF

Preparation Time: 10 minutes   **Cooking Time:** 40 minutes   **Servings: 6**

Ingredients:
- ✓ 2 ½ lb ground tofu
- ✓ Salt and ground black pepper to taste
- ✓ 3 tbsp flaxseed meal
- ✓ 2 large eggs
- ✓ 2 tbsp olive oil

Directions:
- ❖ Preheat the oven to 400 f and grease a loaf pan with cooking spray. Set aside.
- ❖ In a large bowl, combine the tofu, salt, black pepper, and flaxseed meal. Set aside.
- ❖ In a small bowl, whisk the eggs with the olive oil, lemon juice, parsley, oregano, and garlic.
- ❖ our the mixture onto the mix and combine well.

Ingredients:
- ✓ 1 lemon,1 tbsp juiced
- ✓ ¼ cup freshly chopped parsley
- ✓ ¼ cup freshly chopped oregano
- ✓ 4 garlic cloves, minced
- ✓ Lemon slices to garnish

- ❖ Spoon the tofu mixture into the loaf pan and press to fit into the pan
- ❖ Bake in the middle rack of the oven for 30 to 40 minutes.
- ❖ Remove the pan, tilt to drain the meat's liquid, and allow cooling for 5 minutes.
- ❖ Slice, garnish with some lemon slices and serve with braised green beans.

70) VEGAN BACON WRAPPED TOFU WITH BUTTERED SPINACH

Preparation Time: 5 minutes   **Cooking Time:** 20 minutes   **Servings: 4**

Ingredients:
- ✓ For the bacon wrapped tofu:
- ✓ 4 tofu
- ✓ 8 slices vegan bacon
- ✓ Salt and black pepper to taste
- ✓ 2 tbsp olive oil

Directions:
- ❖ For the bacon wrapped tofu:
- ❖ Preheat the oven to 450 f.
- ❖ Wrap each tofu with two vegan bacon slices
- ❖ Season with salt and black pepper, and place on the baking sheet
- ❖ Drizzle with the olive oil and bake in the oven for 15 minutes
- ❖ (Or until the vegan bacon browns and the tofu cooks within)

Ingredients:
- ✓ For the buttered spinach:
- ✓ 2 tbsp butter
- ✓ 1 lb spinach
- ✓ 4 garlic cloves
- ✓ Salt and ground black pepper to taste

- ❖ For the buttered spinach:
- ❖ Meanwhile, melt the butter in a large skillet
- ❖ Add and sauté the spinach and garlic until the leaves wilt, 5 minutes
- ❖ Season with salt and black pepper.
- ❖ Remove the tofu from the oven and serve with the buttered spinach.

71) CAULIFLOWER MIX

Preparation Time: 10 minutes   **Cooking Time:** 25 minutes   **Servings: 4**

Ingredients:
- ✓ 1 pound cauliflower florets
- ✓ 2 tablespoons avocado oil
- ✓ 1 teaspoon nutmeg, ground
- ✓ 1 teaspoon hot paprika

Directions:
- ❖ Spread the cauliflower florets on a baking sheet lined with parchment paper
- ❖ Add the oil, the nutmeg and the other ingredients, toss

Ingredients:
- ✓ 1 tablespoon pumpkin seeds
- ✓ 1 tablespoon chives, chopped
- ✓ A pinch of sea salt and black pepper

- ❖ Bake at 380 degrees F for 25 minutes.
- ❖ Divide the cauliflower mix between plates and serve.

72) BAKED BROCCOLI AND PINE NUTS

Preparation Time: 10 minutes   **Cooking Time:** 30 minutes   **Servings: 4**

Ingredients:
- ✓ 2 tablespoons olive oil
- ✓ 1 pound broccoli florets
- ✓ 1 tablespoon garlic, minced
- ✓ 1 tablespoon pine nuts, toasted

Ingredients:
- ✓ 1 tablespoon lemon juice
- ✓ 2 teaspoons mustard
- ✓ A pinch of salt and black pepper

Directions:
- ❖ In a roasting pan, combine the broccoli with the oil, the garlic
- ❖ Add the other ingredients, toss
- ❖ Bake at 380 degrees F for 30 minutes.
- ❖ Divide everything between plates and serve.

73) CHILI ASPARAGUS

Preparation Time: 10 minutes   **Cooking Time:** 15 minutes   **Servings: 4**

Ingredients:
- ✓ 1 yellow onion, chopped
- ✓ 2 tablespoons olive oil
- ✓ 1 bunch asparagus, trimmed and halved

Ingredients:
- ✓ 2 garlic cloves, minced
- ✓ 1 teaspoon chili powder
- ✓ ¼ cup cilantro, chopped

Directions:
- ❖ Heat up a pan with the oil over medium-high heat
- ❖ Add the onion and the garlic and sauté for 5 minutes.
- ❖ Then the asparagus and the other ingredients, toss
- ❖ Cook for 10 minutes, divide between plates and serve.

74) TOMATO QUINOA

Preparation Time: 10 minutes   **Cooking Time:** 25 minutes   **Servings: 4**

Ingredients:
- ✓ 1 cup quinoa
- ✓ 3 cups chicken stock
- ✓ 1 cup tomatoes, cubed
- ✓ 1 tablespoon parsley, chopped

Ingredients:
- ✓ 1 tablespoon basil, chopped
- ✓ 1 teaspoon turmeric powder
- ✓ A pinch of salt and black pepper

Directions:
- ❖ In a pot, mix the quinoa with the stock, the tomatoes
- ❖ Add the other ingredients, toss
- ❖ Bring to a simmer and cook over medium heat for 25 minutes.
- ❖ Divide everything between plates and serve.

75) CORIANDER BLACK BEANS

Preparation Time: 10 minutes   **Cooking Time:** 20 minutes   **Servings: 4**

Ingredients:
- ✓ 1 tablespoon olive oil
- ✓ 2 cups canned black beans, drained and rinsed
- ✓ 1 green bell pepper, chopped
- ✓ 1 yellow onion, chopped
- ✓ 4 garlic cloves, minced

Ingredients:
- ✓ 1 teaspoon cumin, ground
- ✓ ½ cup chicken stock
- ✓ 1 tablespoon coriander, chopped
- ✓ A pinch of salt and black pepper

Directions:
- ❖ Heat up a pan with the oil over medium heat
- ❖ Add the onion and the garlic and sauté for 5 minutes.
- ❖ Then the black beans and the other ingredients, toss
- ❖ Cook over medium heat for 15 minutes more
- ❖ Divide between plates and serve.

76) GREEN BEANS AND MANGO MIX

Preparation Time: 10 minutes   **Cooking Time:** 20 minutes   **Servings: 4**

Ingredients:
- ✓ 1 pound green beans, trimmed and halved
- ✓ 3 scallions, chopped
- ✓ 1 mango, peeled and cubed
- ✓ 2 tablespoons olive oil

Directions:
- ❖ Heat up a pan with the oil over medium heat
- ❖ Add the scallions and sauté for 2 minutes.

Ingredients:
- ✓ ½ cup veggie stock
- ✓ 1 tablespoon oregano, chopped
- ✓ 1 teaspoon sweet paprika
- ✓ A pinch of salt and black pepper

- ❖ Then the green beans and the other ingredients, toss
- ❖ Cook over medium heat for 18 minutes more
- ❖ Divide between plates and serve.

77) QUINOA WITH OLIVES

Preparation Time: 10 minutes   **Cooking Time:** 30 minutes   **Servings: 4**

Ingredients:
- ✓ 1 yellow onion, chopped
- ✓ 1 tablespoon olive oil
- ✓ 1 cup quinoa
- ✓ 3 cups vegetable stock
- ✓ ½ cup black olives, pitted and halved

Directions:
- ❖ Heat up a pot with the oil over medium heat
- ❖ Add the yellow onion and sauté for 5 minutes.
- ❖ Then the quinoa and the other ingredients except the green onions, stir

Ingredients:
- ✓ 2 green onions, chopped
- ✓ 2 tablespoons coconut aminos
- ✓ 1 teaspoon rosemary, dried

- ❖ Bring to a simmer and cook over medium heat for 25 minutes.
- ❖ Divide the mix between plates
- ❖ Sprinkle the green onions on top and serve.

78) GARLIC ASPARAGUS AND TOMATOES

Preparation Time: 10 minutes   **Cooking Time:** 20 minutes   **Servings: 4**

Ingredients:
- ✓ 1 pound asparagus, trimmed and halved
- ✓ ½ pound cherry tomatoes, halved
- ✓ 2 tablespoons olive oil
- ✓ 1 teaspoon turmeric powder

Directions:
- ❖ Spread the asparagus on a baking sheet lined with parchment paper
- ❖ Add the tomatoes and the other ingredients, toss

Ingredients:
- ✓ 2 tablespoons shallot, chopped
- ✓ A pinch of salt and black pepper
- ✓ 1 tablespoon chives, chopped

- ❖ Cook in the oven at 375 degrees F for 20 minutes.
- ❖ Divide everything between plates and serve

79) HOT CUCUMBER MIX

Preparation Time: 10 minutes   **Cooking Time:** 0 minutes   **Servings: 4**

Ingredients:
- ✓ 1 pound cucumbers, sliced
- ✓ 1 tablespoon olive oil
- ✓ 1 teaspoon chili powder
- ✓ 1 green chili, chopped

Ingredients:
- ✓ 1 garlic clove, minced
- ✓ 1 tablespoon dill, chopped
- ✓ 2 tablespoons lime juice
- ✓ 1 tablespoon balsamic vinegar

Directions:
- ❖ In a bowl, combine the cucumbers with the garlic, the oil
- ❖ Add the other ingredients
- ❖ Toss and serve as a salad.

80) TOMATO SALAD

Preparation Time: 10 minutes   **Cooking Time:** 0 minutes   **Servings: 4**

Ingredients:
- ✓ 1 pound cherry tomatoes, halved
- ✓ 3 scallions, chopped
- ✓ 1 tablespoon olive oil

Ingredients:
- ✓ A pinch of salt and black pepper
- ✓ 1 tablespoon lime juice
- ✓ ¼ cup parsley, chopped

Directions:
- ❖ In a bowl, combine the tomatoes with the scallions
- ❖ Add the other ingredients
- ❖ Toss and serve as a salad.

DESSERT RECIPES

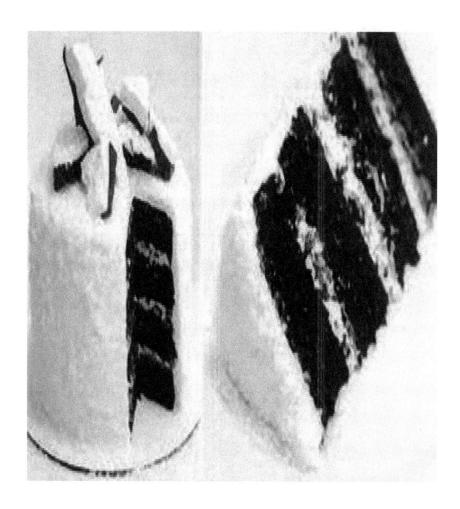

81) CHOCOLATE WATERMELON CUPS

Preparation Time: 2 hours   **Cooking Time:** 0 minutes   **Servings: 4**

Ingredients:
- ✓ 2 cups watermelon, peeled and cubed
- ✓ 1 tablespoon stevia
- ✓ 1 cup coconut cream

Ingredients:
- ✓ 1 tablespoon cocoa powder
- ✓ 1 tablespoon mint, chopped

Directions:
- ❖ In a blender, combine the watermelon with the stevia
- ❖ Add the other ingredients

- ❖ Pulse well, divide into cups
- ❖ Keep in the fridge for 2 hours before serving.

82) VANILLA RASPBERRIES MIX

Preparation Time: 10 minutes   **Cooking Time:** 10 minutes   **Servings: 4**

Ingredients:
- ✓ 1 cup water
- ✓ 1 cup raspberries
- ✓ 3 tablespoons stevia

Ingredients:
- ✓ 1 teaspoon nutmeg, ground
- ✓ ½ teaspoon vanilla extract

Directions:
- ❖ In a pan, combine the raspberries with the water
- ❖ Add the other ingredients

- ❖ Toss, cook over medium heat for 10 minutes
- ❖ Divide into bowls and serve.

83) COCONUT SALAD

Preparation Time: 10 minutes   **Cooking Time:** 0 minutes   **Servings: 6**

Ingredients:
- ✓ 2 cups coconut flesh, unsweetened and shredded
- ✓ ½ cup walnuts, chopped
- ✓ 1 cup blackberries

Ingredients:
- ✓ 1 tablespoon stevia
- ✓ 1 tablespoon coconut oil, melted

Directions:
- ❖ In a bowl, combine the coconut with the walnuts

- ❖ Add the other ingredients:, toss and serve.

84) MINT COOKIES

Preparation Time: 10 minutes   **Cooking Time:** 20 minutes   **Servings: 6**

Ingredients:
- ✓ 2 cups coconut flour
- ✓ 3 tablespoons flaxseed mixed with
- ✓ 4 tablespoons water
- ✓ ½ cup coconut cream

Ingredients:
- ✓ ½ cup coconut oil, melted
- ✓ 3 tablespoons stevia
- ✓ 2 teaspoons mint, dried
- ✓ 2 teaspoons baking soda

Directions:
- ❖ In a bowl, mix the coconut flour with the flaxseed, coconut cream
- ❖ Add the other ingredients, and whisk really well.

- ❖ Shape balls out of this mix, place them on a lined baking sheet, flatten them
- ❖ Introduce in the oven at 370 degrees F
- ❖ Bake for 20 minutes. Serve the cookies cold.

85) MINT AVOCADO BARS

Preparation Time: 10 minutes   **Cooking Time:** 25 minutes   **Servings: 6**

Ingredients:
- ✓ 1 teaspoon almond extract
- ✓ ½ cup coconut oil, melted
- ✓ 2 tablespoons stevia

Directions:
- ❖ In a bowl, combine the coconut oil with the almond extract
- ❖ Add stevia and the other ingredients and whisk well.

Ingredients:
- ✓ 1 avocado, peeled, pitted and mashed
- ✓ 2 cups coconut flour
- ✓ 1 tablespoon cocoa powder

- ❖ Transfer this to baking pan, spread evenly
- ❖ Introduce in the oven and cook at 370 degrees F
- ❖ Bake for 25 minutes. Cool down, cut into bars and serve.

86) COCONUT CHOCOLATE CAKE

Preparation Time: 10 minutes   **Cooking Time:** 30 minutes   **Servings: 12**

Ingredients:
- ✓ 4 tablespoons flaxseed mixed with
- ✓ 5 tablespoons water
- ✓ 1 cup coconut flesh, unsweetened and shredded
- ✓ 1 teaspoon vanilla extract
- ✓ 2 tablespoons cocoa powder

Directions:
- ❖ In a bowl, combine the flaxmeal with the coconut, the vanilla
- ❖ Add the other Ingredients

Ingredients:
- ✓ 1 teaspoon baking soda
- ✓ 2 cups almond flour
- ✓ 4 tablespoons stevia
- ✓ 2 tablespoons lime zest
- ✓ 2 cups coconut cream

- ❖ Whisk well and transfer to a cake pan.
- ❖ Cook the cake at 360 degree F for 30 minutes
- ❖ Cool down and serve.

87) MINT CHOCOLATE CREAM

Preparation Time: 10 minutes   **Cooking Time:** 0 minutes   **Servings: 6**

Ingredients:
- ✓ 1 cup coconut oil, melted
- ✓ 4 tablespoons cocoa powder
- ✓ 1 teaspoon vanilla extract

Directions:
- ❖ In your food processor, combine the coconut oil with the cocoa powder

Ingredients:
- ✓ 1 cup mint, chopped
- ✓ 2 cups coconut cream
- ✓ 4 tablespoons stevia

- ❖ Add the cream and the other ingredients, pulse well
- ❖ Divide into bowls and serve really cold.

88) CRANBERRIES CAKE

Preparation Time: 10 minutes   **Cooking Time:** 30 minutes   **Servings: 6**

Ingredients:
- ✓ 2 cups coconut flour
- ✓ 2 tablespoon coconut oil, melted
- ✓ 3 tablespoons stevia
- ✓ 1 tablespoon cocoa powder, unsweetened
- ✓ 2 tablespoons flaxseed mixed with

Ingredients:
- ✓ 3 tablespoons water
- ✓ 1 cup cranberries
- ✓ 1 cup coconut cream
- ✓ ¼ teaspoon vanilla extract
- ✓ ½ teaspoon baking powder
- ❖ Introduce in the oven
- ❖ Cook at 360 degrees F for 30 minutes.
- ❖ Cool down, slice and serve.

Directions:
- ❖ In a bowl, combine the coconut flour with the coconut oil
- ❖ Add the stevia and the other ingredients, and whisk well.
- ❖ Pour this into a cake pan lined with parchment paper

89) SWEET ZUCCHINI BUNS

Preparation Time: 10 minutes   **Cooking Time:** As per directions   **Servings: 8**

Ingredients:
- ✓ 1 cup almond flour
- ✓ 1/3 cup coconut flesh, unsweetened and shredded
- ✓ 1 cup zucchinis, grated
- ✓ 2 tablespoons stevia
- ✓ 1 teaspoon baking soda

Ingredients:
- ✓ ½ teaspoon cinnamon powder
- ✓ 3 tablespoons flaxseed mixed with
- ✓ 4 tablespoons water
- ✓ 1 cup coconut cream

Directions:
- ❖ In a bowl, mix the almond flour with the coconut flesh, the zucchinis
- ❖ Add the other ingredients
- ❖ Stir well until you obtain a dough, shape 8 buns

- ❖ Arrange them on a baking sheet lined with parchment paper.
- ❖ Introduce in the oven at 350 degrees
- ❖ Bake for 30 minutes. Serve these sweet buns warm.

90) LIME CUSTARD

Preparation Time: 10 minutes   **Cooking Time:** As per directions   **Servings: 6**

Ingredients:
- ✓ 1 pint almond milk
- ✓ 4 tablespoons lime zest, grated
- ✓ 3 tablespoons lime juice

Ingredients:
- ✓ 3 tablespoons flaxseed mixed with
- ✓ 4 tablespoons water tablespoons stevia
- ✓ 2 teaspoons vanilla extract
- ❖ Whisk well and divide into 4 ramekins.
- ❖ Bake in the oven at 360 degrees F for 30 minutes.
- ❖ Cool the custard down and serve.

Directions:
- ❖ In a bowl, combine the almond milk with the lime zest, lime juice
- ❖ Add the other Ingredients

91) CANDIED PECANS

Preparation Time: 60 minutes   **Cooking Time:** As per directions   **Servings: 4**

Ingredients:
- ✓ 6 oz. Whole Pecans
- ✓ ½ cup Aquafaba
- ✓ 1 oz. Palm Sugar

Ingredients:
- ✓ 1 oz. whole Green Cardamom Pods
- ✓ ¼ tsp. Salt
- ✓ 1 tsp. Allspice

Directions:
- ❖ Pre-heat oven to 350°F/180°C.
- ❖ Prepare a baking tray with a piece of parchment paper.
- ❖ Remove the cardamom seeds from the pods
- ❖ Crush the seeds and lay them onto one side of the tray.
- ❖ Chop the sugar or grind it in a food processor.
- ❖ Whisk the aquafaba until frothy

- ❖ Stir in the sugar and salt
- ❖ Fold in the nuts, allspice, cardamom, until everything is coated.
- ❖ Spread the mixture evenly over the baking tray for about 15 minutes
- ❖ Replace it onto the cooling rack.
- ❖ When cooled, pecans can be enjoyed as a topping or as they are.

92) RICE AND CANTALOUPE RAMEKINS

Preparation Time: 10 minutes   **Cooking Time:** 30 minutes   **Servings: 4**

Ingredients:
- ✓ 2 tablespoons flaxseed mixed with
- ✓ 3 tablespoons water
- ✓ 2 cups cauliflower rice, steamed
- ✓ 1 cup coconut cream

Ingredients:
- ✓ 2 tablespoons stevia
- ✓ 1 teaspoon vanilla extract
- ✓ ½ cup cantaloupe, peeled and chopped
- ✓ Cooking spray

Directions:
- ❖ In a bowl, mix the cauliflower rice with the flaxseed
- ❖ Mix and the other Ingredients except the cooking spray and whisk well.

- ❖ Grease 4 ramekins with the cooking spray
- ❖ Divide the rice mix in each and cook at 360 degrees F for 30 minutes.
- ❖ Serve cold.

93) STRAWBERRIES CREAM

Preparation Time: 10 minutes   **Cooking Time:** 0 minutes   **Servings: 2**

Ingredients:
- ✓ 1 cup strawberries, chopped
- ✓ 1 cup coconut cream

Ingredients:
- ✓ 1 tablespoon stevia
- ✓ ½ teaspoon vanilla extract

Directions:
- ❖ In a blender, combine the strawberries with the cream

- ❖ Add the other ingredients
- ❖ Pulse well, divide into cups and serve cold.

94) ALMOND AND CHIA PUDDING

Preparation Time: 10 minutes   **Cooking Time:** 15 minutes   **Servings: 4**

Ingredients:
- ✓ 1 tablespoon lime juice
- ✓ 1 tablespoon lime zest, grated
- ✓ 2 cups almond milk
- ✓ 2 tablespoons almonds, chopped

Directions:
- ❖ In a pan, mix the almond milk with the chia seeds, the almonds
- ❖ Add the other ingredients

Ingredients:
- ✓ 1 teaspoon almond extract
- ✓ ½ cup chia seeds
- ✓ 2 tablespoons stevia

- ❖ Whisk, bring to a simmer
- ❖ Cook over medium heat for 15 minutes.
- ❖ Divide the mix into bowls and serve cold.

95) DATES AND COCOA BOWLS

Preparation Time: 2 hours   **Cooking Time:** 0 minutes   **Servings: 6**

Ingredients:
- ✓ 2 tablespoons avocado oil
- ✓ 1 cup coconut cream
- ✓ 1 teaspoon cocoa powder

Directions:
- ❖ In a bowl, mix the cream with the oil, the cocoa, the cream
- ❖ Add the other ingredients

Ingredients:
- ✓ ½ cup dates, chopped
- ✓ 3 tablespoons stevia

- ❖ Pulse well, divide into cups
- ❖ Keep in the fridge for 2 hours before serving.

96) NUTS AND SEEDS PUDDING

Preparation Time: 10 minutes   **Cooking Time:** 20 minutes   **Servings: 4**

Ingredients:
- ✓ 2 cups cauliflower rice
- ✓ ¼ cup coconut cream
- ✓ 2 cups almond milk
- ✓ 1 teaspoon vanilla extract

Directions:
- ❖ In a pan, combine the cauliflower rice with the cream, the almond milk
- ❖ Add the other ingredients

Ingredients:
- ✓ 3 tablespoons stevia
- ✓ ½ cup walnuts, chopped
- ✓ 1 tablespoon chia seeds
- ✓ Cooking spray
- ❖ Toss, bring to a simmer
- ❖ Cook over medium heat for 20 minutes.
- ❖ Divide into bowls and serve cold.

97) CASHEW FUDGE

Preparation Time: 3 hours   **Cooking Time:** 0 minutes   **Servings: 6**

Ingredients:
- ✓ 1/3 cup cashew butter
- ✓ 1 cup coconut cream
- ✓ ½ cup cashews, soaked for 8 hours and drained

Directions:
- ❖ In a bowl, mix the cashew butter with the cream, the cashews
- ❖ Add the other ingredients and whisk well.

Ingredients:
- ✓ 5 tablespoons lime juice
- ✓ ½ teaspoon lime zest, grated
- ✓ 1 tablespoons stevia

- ❖ Line a muffin tray with parchment paper, scoop 1 tablespoon of the fudge
- ❖ Mix in each of the muffin tins and freeze for 3 hours before serving.

98) LIME BERRIES STEW

Preparation Time: 10 minutes   **Cooking Time:** 20 minutes   **Servings: 6**

Ingredients:
- ✓ Zest of 1 lime, grated
- ✓ Juice of 1 lime
- ✓ 1 pint strawberries, halved

Directions:
- ❖ In a pan, combine the strawberries with the lime juice, the water and stevia

Ingredients:
- ✓ 2 cups water
- ✓ 2 tablespoons stevia

- ❖ Toss, bring to a simmer and cook over medium heat for 20 minutes.
- ❖ Divide the stew into bowls and serve cold.

99) APRICOTS CAKE

Preparation Time: 10 minutes   **Cooking Time:** 30 minutes   **Servings: 8**

Ingredients:
- ✓ ¾ cup stevia
- ✓ 2 cups coconut flour
- ✓ ¼ cup coconut oil, melted
- ✓ ½ cup almond milk
- ✓ 1 teaspoon baking powder

Directions:
- ❖ In a bowl, mix the flour with the coconut oil, the stevia
- ❖ Add the other ingredients
- ❖ Whisk and pour into a cake pan lined with parchment paper.

Ingredients:
- ✓ 2 tablespoons flaxseed mixed with 3 tablespoons water
- ✓ ½ teaspoon vanilla extract
- ✓ Juice of 1 lime
- ✓ 2 cups apricots, chopped

- ❖ Introduce in the oven at 375 degrees F
- ❖ Bake for 30 minutes, cool down, slice and serve.

Preparation Time: 10 minutes   **Cooking Time:** 30 minutes   **Servings: 6**

Ingredients:
- ✓ 2 cups coconut flour
- ✓ 1 cup blueberries
- ✓ 1 cup strawberries, chopped
- ✓ 2 tablespoons almonds, chopped
- ✓ 2 tablespoons walnuts, chopped
- ✓ 3 tablespoons stevia
- ✓ 1 teaspoon almond extract

Directions:

❖ In a bowl, combine the coconut flour with the berries

❖ Add the nuts, stevia and the other ingredients, and whisk well.

Ingredients:
- ✓ 3 tablespoons flaxseed mixed with
- ✓ 4 tablespoons water
- ✓ ½ cup coconut cream
- ✓ 2 tablespoons avocado oil
- ✓ 1 teaspoon baking powder
- ✓ Cooking spray

❖ Grease a cake pan with the cooking spray, pour the cake mix inside

❖ Introduce everything in the oven at 360 degrees F

❖ Bake for 30 minutes. Cool the cake down, slice and serve.

VEGETARIAN DIET FOR KIDS
BREAKFAST RECIPES

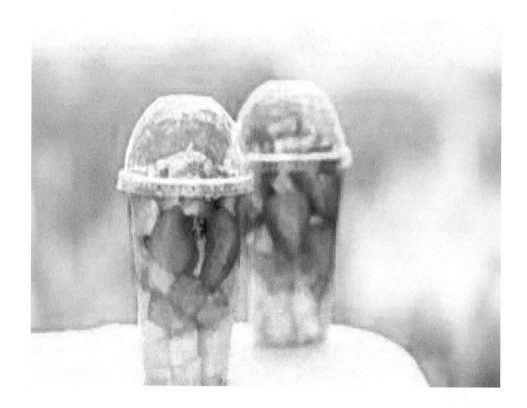

101) BERRIES WITH MASCARPONE ON TOASTED BREAD

Preparation Time: 10 minutes   **Cooking Time:** 0 minute   **Servings: 1**

Ingredients:

- ✓ 1 slice whole-wheat bread
- ✓ 2 tablespoons mascarpone cheese
- ✓ 1/8 cup raspberries

Directions:

- ❖ Spread the cheese on the bread.
- ❖ Top with the berries and chopped mint leaves

Ingredients:

- ✓ 1/8 cup strawberries
- ✓ 1 teaspoon fresh mint leaves

- ❖ Store in food container and refrigerate.
- ❖ Toast in the oven when ready to eat.

102) FRUIT CUP

Preparation Time: 15 minutes   **Cooking Time:** 0 minute   **Servings: 4**

Ingredients:

- ✓ 1 cups melon, sliced
- ✓ 2 cups strawberries, sliced
- ✓ 2 cups grapes, sliced in half
- ✓ 2 cups peaches, sliced
- ✓ 3 tablespoons freshly squeezed lime juice

Directions:

- ❖ Toss the fruits in lime juice, ginger and honey
- ❖ Sprinkle the lime zest on top.

Ingredients:

- ✓ ½ teaspoon ground ginger
- ✓ 1 tablespoon honey
- ✓ 3 teaspoons lime zest
- ✓ ¼ cup coconut flakes, toasted

- ❖ Top with the coconut flakes.

103) OATMEAL WITH BLACK BEANS & CHEDDAR

Preparation Time: 10 minutes   **Cooking Time:** 0 minute   **Servings: 2**

Ingredients:

- ✓ ½ cup rolled oats
- ✓ ¼ cup Vegan yogurt
- ✓ ½ cup almond milk
- ✓ 2 tablespoons seasoned black beans

Directions:

- ❖ Mix all the ingredients except the cilantro in a glass jar with lid.
- ❖ Refrigerate for up to 5 days.

Ingredients:

- ✓ 2 tablespoons Cheddar cheese, shredded
- ✓ 1 stalk scallion, minced
- ✓ 1 tablespoon cilantro, chopped

- ❖ Sprinkle the cilantro on top before serving.

104) BREAKFAST SMOOTHIE

Preparation Time: 10 minutes   **Cooking Time:** 0 minute   **Servings: 2**

Ingredients:

- ✓ ½ cup strawberries
- ✓ ½ cup mango, sliced
- ✓ ½ banana, sliced

Directions:

- ❖ Put all the ingredients in a blender.
- ❖ Pulse until smooth.

Ingredients:

- ✓ ½ cup coconut milk
- ✓ 1 tablespoon cashew butter
- ✓ 1 tablespoon ground chia seeds

- ❖ Refrigerate overnight.

105) YOGURT WITH BEETS & RASPBERRIES

Preparation Time: 5 minutes   **Cooking Time**: 0 minute   **Servings: 1**

Ingredients:
- ✓ 1 cup soy yogurt
- ✓ ½ cup beets, cooked and sliced

Ingredients:
- ✓ 1 tablespoon raspberry jam
- ✓ 1 tablespoon almonds, slivered

Directions:
- ❖ Mix all the ingredients in a glass jar with lid.
- ❖ Sprinkle the almonds on top.

- ❖ Refrigerate for up to 2 days.

106) CURRY OATMEAL

Preparation Time: 10 minutes   **Cooking Time**: 0 minute   **Servings: 3**

Ingredients:
- ✓ 1 tablespoon pure peanut butter
- ✓ ½ cup rolled oats
- ✓ ½ cup coconut milk
- ✓ ½ teaspoon curry powder

Ingredients:
- ✓ 1 teaspoon tamari
- ✓ ¼ cup cooked kale
- ✓ 1 tablespoon cilantro, chopped
- ✓ 2 tablespoons tomatoes, chopped

Directions:
- ❖ Mix all the ingredients except the kale, cilantro and tomatoes
- ❖ Transfer to a glass jar with lid.

- ❖ Refrigerate for up to 5 days.
- ❖ Top with the remaining ingredients when ready to serve.

107) FIG & CHEESE OATMEAL

Preparation Time: 10 minutes   **Cooking Time**: 0 minute   **Servings: 1**

Ingredients:
- ✓ ½ cup water
- ✓ ½ cup rolled oats Pinch salt
- ✓ 2 tablespoons dried figs, sliced

Ingredients:
- ✓ 2 tablespoons ricotta cheese
- ✓ 2 teaspoons agave syrup
- ✓ 1 tablespoon almonds, toasted and sliced

Directions:
- ❖ Put the water, oats and salt in a glass jar with lid.
- ❖ Shake to blend well. Refrigerate for up to 5 days.

- ❖ Top with the remaining ingredients when ready to serve.

108) PUMPKIN OATS

Preparation Time: 10 minutes   **Cooking Time**: 0 minute   **Servings: 1**

Ingredients:
- ✓ ½ cup rolled oats
- ✓ ½ cup almond milk
- ✓ ¼ cup ricotta cheese
- ✓ 2 tablespoons pumpkin puree

Ingredients:
- ✓ 1 tablespoon maple syrup
- ✓ ¼ teaspoon vanilla
- ✓ 1/8 teaspoon ground nutmeg

Directions:
- ❖ Combine all the ingredients in a glass jar with lid

- ❖ Refrigerate for up to 5 days.

109) SWEET POTATO TOASTS

Preparation Time: 10 minutes   **Cooking Time:** 10 minutes   **Servings: 2**

Ingredients:

- ✓ 2 large sweet potatoes, sliced into ¼ inch thick slices
- ✓ 1 tablespoon avocado oil
- ✓ 1 teaspoon salt

Directions:

- ❖ Preheat your oven to 425 degrees F.
- ❖ Cover a baking sheet with parchment paper.
- ❖ Rub the potato slices with oil and salt

Ingredients:

- ✓ ½ cup guacamole
- ✓ ½ cup tomatoes, sliced

- ❖ Place them on a baking sheet. Bake for 5 minutes in the oven
- ❖ Then flip and bake again for 5 minutes
- ❖ Top the baked slices with guacamole and tomatoes. Serve.

110) TOFU SCRAMBLE TACOS

Preparation Time: 10 minutes   **Cooking Time:** 10 minutes   **Servings: 4**

Ingredients:

- ✓ 1 package tofu
- ✓ ¼ cup nutritional yeast
- ✓ 2 teaspoons garlic powder
- ✓ 2 teaspoons cumin
- ✓ 2 teaspoons chili powder

Directions:

- ❖ In a pan, add avocado oil and tofu.
- ❖ Sauté and crumble the tofu on medium heat

Ingredients:

- ✓ ½ teaspoon turmeric
- ✓ 1 teaspoon salt
- ✓ ½ teaspoon pepper
- ✓ 1 tablespoon avocado oil Warm corn tortillas

- ❖ Stir in all the remaining spices and yeast.
- ❖ Mix and cook for 2 minutes. Serve on tortillas.

111) TASTY OATMEAL AND CARROT CAKE

Preparation Time: 10 minutes   **Cooking Time:** 10 minutes   **Servings: 1**

Ingredients:

- ✓ 1 cup, water
- ✓ ½ teaspoon, cinnamon
- ✓ 1 cup, rolled oats
- ✓ Salt
- ✓ ¼ cup, raisins
- ✓ ½ cup, shredded carrots
- ✓ 1 cup, non-dairy milk

Directions:

- ❖ Put a small pot on low heat and bring the non-dairy milk, oats, and water to a simmer.
- ❖ Now, add the carrots, vanilla extract, raisins, salt, cinnamon and allspice
- ❖ Simmer all of the ingredients, but do not forget to stir them

Ingredients:

- ✓ ¼ teaspoon, allspice
- ✓ ½ teaspoon, vanilla extract
  Toppings:
- ✓ ¼ cup, chopped walnuts
- ✓ 2 tablespoons, maple syrup
- ✓ 2 tablespoons, shredded coconut

- ❖ They are ready when the liquid is fully absorbed into all of the ingredients
- ❖ (In about 7-10 minutes).
- ❖ Transfer the thickened dish to bowls
- ❖ Drizzle some maple syrup on top or top them with coconut or walnuts.

112) ONION & MUSHROOM TART WITH A NICE BROWN RICE CRUST

Preparation Time: 10 minutes **Cooking Time**: 55 minutes **Servings: 1**

Ingredients:

- ✓ 1 ½ pounds, mushrooms, button, portabella
- ✓ 1 cup, short-grain brown rice
- ✓ 2 ¼ cups, water
- ✓ ½ teaspoon, ground black pepper
- ✓ 2 teaspoons, herbal spice blend
- ✓ 1 sweet large onion
- ✓ 7 ounces, extra-firm tofu

Directions:

- ❖ Cook the brown rice and put it aside for later use.
- ❖ Slice the onions into thin strips and sauté them in water until they are soft.
- ❖ Then, add the molasses, and cook them for a few minutes.
- ❖ Next, sauté the mushrooms in water with the herbal spice blend
- ❖ Once the mushrooms are cooked and they are soft
- ❖ Add the white wine or sherry. Cook everything for a few more minutes.
- ❖ In a blender, combine milk, tofu, arrowroot, turmeric
- ❖ Add onion powder till you have a smooth mixture
- ❖ On a pie plate, create a layer of rice, spreading evenly to form a crust
- ❖ The rice should be warm and not cold
- ❖ It will be easy to work with warm rice

Ingredients:

- ✓ 1 cup, plain non-dairy milk
- ✓ 2 teaspoons, onion powder
- ✓ 2 teaspoons, low-sodium soy
- ✓ 1 teaspoon, molasses
- ✓ ¼ teaspoon, ground turmeric
- ✓ ¼ cup, white wine
- ✓ ¼ cup, tapioca
- ❖ Use a pastry roller to get an even crust
- ❖ With your fingers, gently press the sides.
- ❖ Take half of the tofu mixture and the mushrooms
- ❖ Spoon them over the tart dish. Smooth the level with your spoon.
- ❖ Now, top the layer with onions followed by the tofu mixture
- ❖ Smooth the surface again with your spoon.
- ❖ Sprinkle some black pepper on top
- ❖ Bake the pie at 350o F for about 45 minutes
- ❖ Toward the end, cover it loosely with tin foil
- ❖ This will help the crust to remain moist.
- ❖ Allow the pie crust to cool down, so that you can slice it

113) PERFECT BREAKFAST SHAKE

Preparation Time: 5 minutes **Cooking Time**: 0 minutes **Servings: 2**

Ingredients:

- ✓ 1 tablespoons, raw cacao powder
- ✓ 1 cup, almond milk

Directions:

- ❖ Use a powerful blender to combine all the ingredients
- ❖ Process everything until you have a smooth shake.

Ingredients:

- ✓ 2 frozen bananas
- ✓ 3 tablespoons, natural peanut butter
- ❖ Enjoy a hearty shake to kickstart your day.

114)   BEET GAZPACHO

Preparation Time: 10 minutes   **Cooking Time:** 2 minutes   **Servings: 4**

Ingredients:

- ½ large bunch young beets with stems, roots and leaves
- 2 small cloves garlic, peeled
- Salt to taste
- Pepper to taste
- ½ teaspoon liquid stevia
- 1 glass coconut milk kefir
- 1 teaspoon chopped dill

Ingredients:

- ½ tablespoon canola oil
- 1 small red onion, chopped
- 1 tablespoon apple cider vinegar
- 2 cups vegetable broth or water
- 1 tablespoon chopped chives
- 1 scallion, sliced
- Roasted baby potatoes

Directions:

- Cut the roots and stems of the beets into small pieces
- Thinly slice the beet greens.
- Place a saucepan over medium heat
- Add oil. When the oil is heated, add onion and garlic
- Cook until onion turns translucent.
- Stir in the beets, roots and stem and cook for a minute.
- Add broth, salt and water and cover with a lid. Simmer until tender.

- Then stevia and vinegar and mix well
- Taste and adjust the stevia and vinegar if required.
- Turn off the heat. Blend with an immersion blender until smooth.
- Place the saucepan back over it
- When it begins to boil, add beet greens and cook for a minute
- Turn off the heat. Cool completely. Chill if desired
- Add rest of the ingredients and stir.
- Serve in bowls with roasted potatoes if desired

115)   VEGETABLE RICE

Preparation Time: 7 minutes   **Cooking Time:** 15 minutes   **Servings: 4**

Ingredients:

- ½ cup brown rice, rinsed
- 1 cup water
- ½ teaspoon dried basil
- 1 small onion, chopped
- 2 tablespoons raisins
- 5 ounces frozen peas, thawed
- ½ cup pecan halves, toasted

Ingredients:

- 1 medium carrot, cut into matchsticks
- 4 green onions, cut into 1-inch pieces
- 1 tablespoon olive oil
- ½ teaspoon salt or to taste
- ½ teaspoon crushed red chili flakes or to taste
- Ground pepper or to taste

Directions:

- Place a small saucepan with water over medium heat
- When it begins to boil, add rice and basil. Stir.
- When it again begins to boil, lower the heat and cover with a lid
- Cook for 15 minutes until all the water is absorbed and rice is cooked
- Add more water if you think the rice is not cooked well.

- Meanwhile, place a skillet over medium high heat
- Then carrots, raisins and onions
- Sauté until the vegetables are crisp as well as tender.
- Stir in the peas, salt, pepper and chili flakes
- Add pecans and rice and stir.Serve.

116) AVOCADO WITH HALLOUMI CHEESE

Preparation Time: 10 minutes   **Cooking Time**: 15 minutes   **Servings: 4**

Ingredients:
- ✓ 1 avocado
- ✓ 140 g halloumi cheese
- ✓ 1 teaspoon butter for frying
- ✓ 1 tablespoon of olive oil
- ✓ 1/4 cup sour cream

Ingredients:
- ✓ ¼ fresh cucumber
- ✓ 1 tbsp pistachio nuts
- ✓ salt and pepper
- ✓ ¼ lemon (optional)

Directions:
- ❖ Halloumi cheese cut into slices, heat butter in a frying pan
- ❖ Fry the cheese until golden brown.
- ❖ While the cheese is frying, cut the avocado and remove the stone.
- ❖ Cut the cucumbers into sticks and place with avocado on a plate
- ❖ Sprinkle with lemon juice, olive oil and sprinkle with salt and pepper.
- ❖ Serve with fried cheese and sour cream.

117) VEGETARIAN PIZZA RECIPE

Preparation Time: 10 minutes   **Cooking Time**: 30 minutes   **Servings: 4**

Ingredients:
- ✓ Cake Products:
- ✓ 2 eggs
- ✓ ½ cup mayonnaise
- ✓ ¾ cup of almond flour
- ✓ 1 tablespoon of plantain husk
- ✓ 1 teaspoon of baking powder
- ✓ ½ tsp salt
- ✓ Products-Extras:

Ingredients:
- ✓ 50-60 g mushrooms
- ✓ 1 tablespoon of green pesto
- ✓ 2 tablespoons of olive oil
- ✓ ½ cup 18% cream
- ✓ ¾ cup grated cheese
- ✓ Salt and pepper
- ✓ Arugula

Directions:
- ❖ Preheat to 175 ° C in the oven.
- ❖ Combine well the eggs and mayonnaise
- ❖ Add to the dough the remaining ingredients
- ❖ Combine and wait for 5 minutes.
- ❖ Then add on your hands a few drops of oil and evenly
- ❖ Spread the dough on a baking tray lined with baking paper
- ❖ The thickness should be no more than 1 cm.
- ❖ Bake until the dough starts to brown lightly for 10 minutes
- ❖ Clear from the oven and let it cool down
- ❖ Cut the mushrooms in thin slices at this moment.
- ❖ Put the cream on the cooled cake and add oil and spices to the pesto.
- ❖ Sprinkle with the aged cheese and finish with the mushrooms
- ❖ Place the pizza 5-10 minutes in the oven until the cheese is dissolved
- ❖ Serve with salad from the rocket.

118) CHILI SPINACH AND ZUCCHINI PAN

Preparation Time: 5 minutes   **Cooking Time**: 15 minutes   **Servings: 4**

Ingredients:
- ✓ 1 pound baby spinach
- ✓ 1 tablespoons olive oil
- ✓ 2 zucchinis, sliced
- ✓ 1 tomato, cubed
- ✓ 2 shallots, chopped

Ingredients:
- ✓ 1 tablespoon lime juice
- ✓ 2 garlic cloves, minced
- ✓ 2 teaspoons red chili flakes
- ✓ 1 teaspoon chili powder
- ✓ Salt and black pepper to the taste

Directions:
- ❖ Heat up a pan with the oil over medium heat
- ❖ Add the shallots, garlic, chili powder and chili flakes
- ❖ Stir and sauté for 5 minutes.
- ❖ Add the spinach, zucchinis and the other ingredients, toss
- ❖ Cook over medium heat for 10 minutes more
- ❖ Divide into bowls and serve for breakfast.

119) BASIL TOMATO AND CABBAGE BOWLS

Preparation Time: 5 minutes   **Cooking Time:** 0 minutes   **Servings: 4**

Ingredients:

- ✓ 1 pound cherry tomatoes, halved
- ✓ 1 cup red cabbage, shredded
- ✓ 2 tablespoons balsamic vinegar
- ✓ 2 shallots, chopped

Directions:

- ❖ In a bowl, combine the cabbage with the tomatoes and the other ingredients

Ingredients:

- ✓ 1 tablespoon avocado oil
- ✓ Salt and black pepper to the taste
- ✓ 1 tablespoon basil, chopped

- ❖ Toss and serve for breakfast.

120) SPINACH AND ZUCCHINI HASH

Preparation Time: 5 minutes   **Cooking Time:** 15 minutes   **Servings: 4**

Ingredients:

- ✓ 2 zucchinis, cubed
- ✓ 2 cups baby spinach
- ✓ A pinch of salt and black pepper
- ✓ 1 tablespoon olive oil

Directions:

- ❖ Heat up a pan with the oil over medium heat
- ❖ Add the zucchinis and the chili powder, stir and cook for 5 minutes.
- ❖ Then the rest of the ingredients, toss

Ingredients:

- ✓ 1 teaspoon chili powder
- ✓ 1 teaspoon rosemary, dried
- ✓ ½ cup coconut cream
- ✓ 1 tablespoon chives, chopped

- ❖ Cook the mix for 10 minutes more, divide between plates
- ❖ Serve fro breakfast.

LUNCH RECIPES

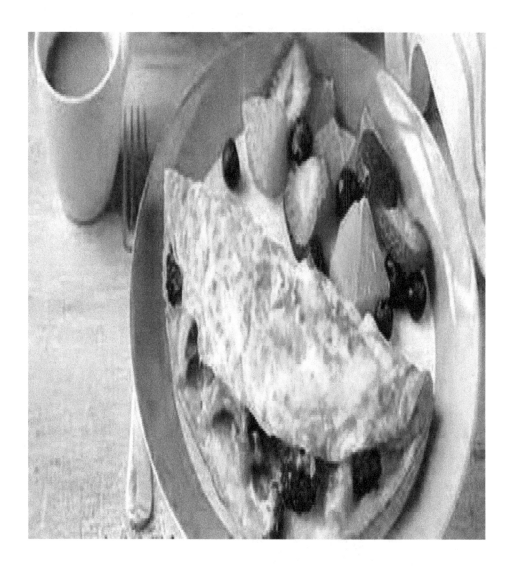

121) RADISH HASH BROWNS

Preparation Time: 10 minutes   **Cooking Time**: 10 minutes   **Servings**: 4

Ingredients:

- ✓ 2 shallots, peeled, sliced
- ✓ ¼ teaspoon thyme
- ✓ ¼ teaspoon paprika
- ✓ 1 organic egg
- ✓ 1 tablespoon coconut flour

Ingredients:

- ✓ 2-ounces cheddar cheese
- ✓ 1 lb. radishes, shredded
- ✓ ¼ teaspoon pepper
- ✓ ¼ teaspoon sea salt

Directions:

- ❖ Add Ingredients into a mixing bowl, except for the butter and mix well.
- ❖ Melt the butter in a pan over medium heat

- ❖ Then a scoop of mixture into the pan and fry until lightly browned on both sides
- ❖ Serve and enjoy!

122) MASHED TURNIPS

Preparation Time: 5 minutes   **Cooking Time:** 20 minutes   **Servings:** 4

Ingredients:

- ✓ 3 cups turnip, diced
- ✓ 2 garlic cloves, minced
- ✓ ¼ cup heavy cream

Ingredients:

- ✓ 3 tablespoons butter, melted
- ✓ Pepper and salt to taste

Directions:

- ❖ Bring your turnip to a boil in a saucepan over medium heat
- ❖ Cook for about 20 minutes
- ❖ Then drain turnips and mash until smooth

- ❖ Add butter, garlic, heavy cream, pepper, and salt
- ❖ Mix well. Serve warm and enjoy!

123) CREAMY COCONUT CURRY

Preparation Time: 15 minutes   **Cooking Time:** 30 minutes   **Servings:** 4

Ingredients:

- ✓ 1 teaspoon garlic, minced
- ✓ 1 teaspoon ginger, minced
- ✓ 2 teaspoons soy sauce
- ✓ 1 tablespoon red curry paste
- ✓ 1 cup broccoli florets

Ingredients:

- ✓ 1 handful spinach
- ✓ ¼ of an onion, sliced
- ✓ ½ cup coconut cream
- ✓ 4 tablespoons coconut oil

Directions:

- ❖ In a saucepan over medium-high heat, heat your coconut oil
- ❖ Add your onion to the pan and cook until softened
- ❖ Then garlic and cook until lightly browned
- ❖ Reduce heat to medium-low, adding broccoli, stir well

- ❖ Cook for about 20 minutes then add the curry paste and stir
- ❖ Join also spinach over broccoli and cook until wilted
- ❖ Add soy sauce, ginger and coconut cream, and stir
- ❖ Simmer for an additional 10 minutes. Serve hot and enjoy!

124) BROCCOLI OMELET

Preparation Time: 10 minutes   **Cooking Time:** 10 minutes   **Servings: 2**

Ingredients:

- ✓ 1 tablespoon extra-virgin olive oil
- ✓ 1 tablespoon parsley, chopped
- ✓ 1 cup broccoli, cooked, chopped

Directions:

- ❖ In a mixing bowl beat eggs with salt and pepper
- ❖ Add broccoli to egg mixture
- ❖ Heat the olive oil in a pan over medium heat

Ingredients:

- ✓ 4 eggs, organic
- ✓ ½ teaspoon sea salt
- ✓ ¼ teaspoon pepper

- ❖ Pour your broccoli and eggs mixture into the pan and cook until set
- ❖ Flip and cook other side until lightly browned
- ❖ Garnish with chopped parsley. Serve and joy!

125) TOMATO SOUP

Preparation Time: 10 minutes   **Cooking Time:** 20 minutes   **Servings: 4**

Ingredients:

- ✓ 2 tablespoons tomato paste
- ✓ 1 tablespoon garlic, minced
- ✓ 1 tablespoon extra-virgin olive oil
- ✓ 4 cups vegetable broth, low-sodium
- ✓ ½ teaspoon thyme, chopped, fresh
- ✓ 1 tablespoon basil, fresh, chopped

Directions:

- ❖ In the saucepan heat your oil over medium heat
- ❖ Add bell pepper, garlic, onion, and tomatoes, sauté for 10 minutes
- ❖ Then remaining Ingredients and stir to combine
- ❖ Increase the heat to high and bring to a boil

Ingredients:

- ✓ 1 teaspoon oregano, fresh, chopped
- ✓ 1 cup onion, chopped
- ✓ 1 cup red bell pepper, chopped
- ✓ 3 cups tomatoes, peeled, seeded, chopped
- ✓ ¼ teaspoon pepper

- ❖ Reduce heat to low and place a lid on the pan
- ❖ Simmer for 10 minutes. Remove from heat
- ❖ Puree the soup using a blender until smooth
- ❖ Serve and enjoy!

126) TOFU SCRAMBLE

Preparation Time: 10 minutes   **Cooking Time:** 10 minutes   **Servings: 4**

Ingredients:

- ✓ 1 garlic clove, minced
- ✓ 1 cup mushrooms, sliced
- ✓ ½ teaspoon turmeric
- ✓ ½ teaspoon pepper
- ✓ ½ teaspoon sea salt

Directions:

- ❖ Heat a pan over medium heat, adding mushrooms, tomato
- ❖ Then onion, garlic and bell pepper
- ❖ Sauté veggies for 5 minutes

Ingredients:

- ✓ 1 small onion, diced
- ✓ 1 tomato, diced
- ✓ 1 bell pepper, diced
- ✓ 1 lb. tofu, firm, drained

- ❖ Crumble the tofu into pan over the veggies
- ❖ Add pepper, turmeric, sea salt and stir well
- ❖ Cook tofu for 5 minutes. Serve and enjoy!

127)   MASHED CAULIFLOWER

Preparation Time: 10 minutes   **Cooking Time:** 15 minutes   **Servings: 6**

Ingredients:

- ✓   2 tablespoons milk
- ✓   4 tablespoons butter
- ✓   2 cauliflower heads, cut into florets
- ✓   ½ teaspoon onion powder

Ingredients:

- ✓   ½ teaspoon garlic powder
- ✓   ½ teaspoon sea salt
- ✓   ½ teaspoon pepper

Directions:

- ❖   Add your cauliflower to a saucepan filled with enough water to cover the cauliflower
- ❖   Cook cauliflower over medium heat for 15 minutes
- ❖   Drain your cauliflower florets and place it in a mixing bowl.

- ❖   Add remaining ingredients to the bowl.
- ❖   Use a blender blend until smooth. Serve and enjoy!

128)   ROASTED CAULIFLOWER

Preparation Time: 10 minutes   **Cooking Time:** 30 minutes   **Servings: 4**

Ingredients:

- ✓   1 cauliflower head, cut into florets
- ✓   2 tablespoons fresh sage, chopped

Ingredients:

- ✓   1 garlic clove, minced
- ✓   1 tablespoon extra-virgin olive oil

Directions:

- ❖   Preheat your oven to 400˚Fahrenheit
- ❖   Coat a baking tray with cooking spray
- ❖   Spread the cauliflower florets on prepared baking tray
- ❖   Bake cauliflower in the oven for 30 minutes

- ❖   Meanwhile, sauté garlic in a pan with one tablespoon of olive oil
- ❖   Remove from heat and set aside.
- ❖   Add cauliflower, garlic, and sage to a bowl and toss to mix. Serve and enjoy!

129)   CREAMY ONION SOUP

Preparation Time: 15 minutes   **Cooking Time:** 25 minutes   **Servings: 4**

Ingredients:

- ✓   1 shallot, sliced
- ✓   Sea salt
- ✓   1 ½ tablespoons extra-virgin olive oil
- ✓   1 leek, sliced

Ingredients:

- ✓   1 garlic clove, chopped
- ✓   4 cups vegetable stock
- ✓   1 onion, sliced

Directions:

- ❖   Add the olive oil and vegetable stock into a large saucepan over medium heat
- ❖   Bring to a boil. add the remaining ingredients and stir
- ❖   Cover and simmer for 25 minutes

- ❖   Puree your soup using a blender until smooth
- ❖   Serve warm and enjoy!

130) BAKED ZUCCHINI EGGPLANT WITH CHEESE

Preparation Time: 15 minutes   **Cooking Time:** 35 minutes   **Servings: 6**

Ingredients:

- ✓ 3 ounces Parmesan cheese, grated
- ✓ 3 medium zucchinis, sliced
- ✓ 1 tablespoon extra-virgin olive oil
- ✓ 1 medium eggplant, sliced
- ✓ 1 cup cherry tomatoes, halved

Ingredients:

- ✓ ¼ cup parsley, chopped
- ✓ ¼ cup basil, chopped
- ✓ 4 garlic cloves, minced
- ✓ ¼ teaspoon sea salt
- ✓ ¼ teaspoon pepper

Directions:

- ❖ Preheat your oven to 350°Fahrenheit
- ❖ Spray a baking dish with cooking spray
- ❖ In a mixing bowl, add eggplant, cherry tomatoes, zucchini
- ❖ Then olive oil, cheese, basil, garlic, salt, and pepper, toss to mix
- ❖ Transfer eggplant mixture to baking dish
- ❖ Place into preheated oven to bake for 35 minutes
- ❖ Garnish with chopped parsley. Serve and enjoy!

131) VEGETABLE CHAR SIU

Preparation Time: 5 min   **Cooking Time:** 15 min   **Servings: 4**

Ingredients:

- ✓ 100 grams Raw Jackfruit, deseeded and rinsed
- ✓ 100 grams Cucumbers, cut into thin strips
- ✓ 50 grams Red Bell Pepper, cut into thin strips
- ✓ 2 cloves Garlic, minced

Ingredients:

- ✓ 1 Shallot, minced
- ✓ ¼ cup Char Siu Sauce
- ✓ ¼ cup Water
- ✓ 2 tbsp Peanut Oil

Directions:

- ❖ Heat peanut oil in a pan.
- ❖ Add jackfruit and stir until slightly brown.
- ❖ Then garlic and shallots and sautee until aromatic.
- ❖ Join also water and char siu sauce
- ❖ Simmer until jackfruit is tender.
- ❖ Shred jackfruit with forks.
- ❖ Toss in cucumbers and bell peppers.

132) SOY CHORIZO

Preparation Time: 5 min   **Cooking Time:** 15 min   **Servings: 6**

Ingredients:

- ✓ 500 grams Firm Tofu, pressed and drained
- ✓ ¼ cup Soy Sauce
- ✓ ¼ cup Red Wine Vinegar
- ✓ ¼ cup Tomato Paste
- ✓ 1 tsp Paprika
- ✓ 1 tsp Chili Powder
- ✓ 1 tsp Garlic Powder

Ingredients:

- ✓ ½ tsp Onion Powder
- ✓ 1 tsp Cumin Powder
- ✓ ½ tsp Black Pepper
- ✓ ½ tsp Salt
- ✓ ¼ cup Olive Oil

Directions:

- ❖ Crumble tofu in a bowl. Mix in all Ingredients except for the olive oil.
- ❖ Heat olive oil in a non-stick pan.
- ❖ Add tofu mix and stir for 10-15 minutes.
- ❖ Serve in tacos, wraps, burritos, or rice bowls.

133) VIETNAMESE "VERMICELLI" SALAD

Preparation Time: 5 min   **Cooking Time:** As direction   **Servings: 4**

Ingredients:

- ✓ 100 grams Carrot, sliced into thin strips
- ✓ 200 grams Cucumbers, spiralized
- ✓ 2 tbsp Roasted Peanuts, roughly chopped
- ✓ ¼ cup Fresh Mint, chopped
- ✓ ¼ cup Fresh Cilantro, chopped
- ✓ 1 tbsp Stevia

Ingredients:

- ✓ 2 tbsp Fresh Lime Juice
- ✓ 1 tbsp Vegan Fish Sauce
- ✓ 2 cloves Garlic, minced
- ✓ 1 Green Chili, deseeded and minced
- ✓ 2 tbsp Sesame Oil

Directions:

- ❖ Whisk together sugar, lime juice, sesame oil, fish sauce
- ❖ Then minced garlic, and chopped chili. Set aside.
- ❖ In a bowl, toss together cucumbers, carrots, cucumbers, peanuts
- ❖ Add mint, cilantro, and prepared dressing.
- ❖ Serve chilled.

134) CREAMY ZUCCHINI QUICHE

Preparation Time: 120 minutes   **Cooking Time:** As per dierections   **Servings: 8**

Ingredients:

- ✓ 2 lbs zucchini, thinly sliced
- ✓ 1 1/2 cup almond milk
- ✓ 2 large eggs

Ingredients:

- ✓ 2 cups cheddar cheese, shredded
- ✓ Pepper
- ✓ Salt

Directions:

- ❖ Preheat the oven to 375 F.
- ❖ Season zucchini with pepper and salt and set aside for 30 minutes.
- ❖ In a large bowl, beat eggs with almond milk, pepper, and salt.
- ❖ Add shredded cheddar cheese and stir well.
- ❖ Spray quiche pan with cooking spray
- ❖ Arrange zucchini slices in quiche pan.
- ❖ Pour egg and milk mixture over zucchini the sprinkle shredded cheese.
- ❖ Bake in preheated oven for 60 minutes
- ❖ (Or until quiche is lightly golden brown)
- ❖ Serve warm and enjoy.

135) SIMPLE GARLIC CAULIFLOWER COUSCOUS

Preparation Time: 30 minutes   **Cooking Time:** As per dierections   **Servings: 3**

Ingredients:

- ✓ 1 medium cauliflower head, cut into florets
- ✓ 2 tsp parsley, dried

Ingredients:

- ✓ 2 tsp garlic, dried Salt

Directions:

- ❖ Add cauliflower florets into the food processor
- ❖ Process until it looks like couscous.
- ❖ Heat large pan over medium-low heat.
- ❖ Then cauliflower couscous, parsley, and garlic in the pan
- ❖ Cook until softened.
- ❖ Stir well and season with salt.
- ❖ Serve and enjoy.

136) GLUTEN FREE ASPARAGUS QUICHE

Preparation Time: 1 h 10 minutes   **Cooking Time:** As directions   **Servings: 6**

Ingredients:

- ✓ 5 eggs, beaten
- ✓ 1 cup Swiss cheese, shredded
- ✓ 1/4 tsp thyme
- ✓ 1/4 tsp white pepper

Directions:

- ❖ Preheat the oven to 350 F.
- ❖ Spray a quiche dish with cooking spray and set aside.
- ❖ In a bowl, beat together eggs, thyme, white pepper, almond milk, and salt.
- ❖ Arrange asparagus in prepared quiche dish

Ingredients:

- ✓ 1 cup almond milk
- ✓ 15 asparagus spears, cut woody ends and cut asparagus in half
- ✓ 1/4 tsp salt
- ❖ Then pour egg mixture over asparagus.
- ❖ Sprinkle shredded cheese all over asparagus and egg mixture.
- ❖ Place in preheated oven and bake for 60 minutes.
- ❖ Cut quiche into slices and serve.

137) MINI VEGETABLE QUICHE

Preparation Time: 30 minutes   **Cooking Time:** As directions   **Servings: 12**

Ingredients:

- ✓ 7 eggs
- ✓ 1/4 cup onion, chopped
- ✓ 1/4 cup mushroom, diced

Directions:

- ❖ Line muffin cups with aluminum foil cups set aside.
- ❖ Add all Ingredients into the large bowl and beat lightly to combine.

Ingredients:

- ✓ 1/4 cup bell pepper, diced
- ✓ 3/4 cup cheddar cheese, shredded
- ✓ 10 oz frozen spinach, chopped
- ❖ Pour egg mixture into the prepared muffin tray.
- ❖ Bake at 350 F for 20 minutes.
- ❖ Serve warm and enjoy.

138) SIMPLE ROASTED RADISHES

Preparation Time: 45 minutes   **Cooking Time:** As directions   **Servings: 2**

Ingredients:

- ✓ 3 cups radish, clean and halved
- ✓ 3 tbsp olive oil

Directions:

- ❖ Preheat the oven to 425 F.
- ❖ Add radishes, salt, peppercorns, rosemary
- ❖ Then 2 tablespoons of olive oil in a bowl and toss well.
- ❖ Pour radishes mixture into the baking sheet

Ingredients:

- ✓ 2 tbsp fresh rosemary, chopped
- ✓ 10 black peppercorns, crushed 2 tsp sea salt
- ❖ Bake in preheated oven for 30 minutes.
- ❖ Heat remaining olive oil in a pan over medium heat.
- ❖ Add baked radishes in the pan and sauté for 2 minutes.
- ❖ Serve immediately and enjoy.

139) COCONUT BROCCOLI CHEESE LOAF

Preparation Time: 35 minutes   **Cooking Time:** As directions   **Servings: 5**

Ingredients:

- ✓ 5 eggs, lightly beaten
- ✓ 2 tsp baking powder
- ✓ 3 1/1 tbsp coconut flour

Directions:

- ❖ Preheat the oven to 350 F.
- ❖ Spray a loaf pan with cooking spray and set aside.
- ❖ Add all Ingredients into the bowl and mix well.

Ingredients:

- ✓ 3/4 cup broccoli florets, chopped
- ✓ 1 cup cheddar cheese, shredded
- ✓ 1 tsp salt
- ❖ Pour egg mixture into the prepared loaf pan
- ❖ Bake in preheated oven for 30 minutes.
- ❖ Cut loaf into the slices and serve.

140) GREEN PARSLEY BROCCOLI CAULIFLOWER PUREE

Preparation Time: 35 minutes   **Cooking Time:** As directions   **Servings: 4**

Ingredients:

- ✓ 1 1/3 small broccoli, cut into florets
- ✓ 4 tbsp fresh parsley
- ✓ 1 small cauliflower, cut into florets

Directions:

- ❖ Add cauliflower and broccoli in steamer and steam for 15 minutes.

Ingredients:

- ✓ 2 cups vegetable broth
- ✓ 4 tbsp butter
- ✓ 1 tsp sea salt
- ❖ Then steamed cauliflower and broccoli in a blender with butter, broth, and parsley
- ❖ Blend until smooth. Season puree with salt and serve.

SNACK RECIPES

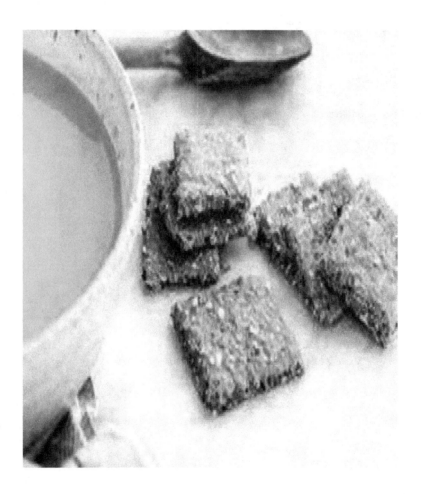

141) JICAMA AND GUACAMOLE

Preparation Time: 15 minutes   **Cooking Time:** 0 minutes   **Servings: 4**

Ingredients:
- ✓ Juice of 1 lime, or 1 tablespoon prepared lime juice
- ✓ 2 hass avocados, peeled, pits removed, and cut into cubes
- ✓ ½ teaspoon sea salt
- ✓ ½ red onion, minced

Ingredients:
- ✓ 1 garlic clove, minced
- ✓ ¼ cup chopped cilantro (optional
- ✓ 1 jicama bulb, peeled and cut into matchsticks

Directions:
- ❖ In a medium bowl, squeeze the lime juice over the top of the avocado and sprinkle with salt.
- ❖ Lightly mash the avocado with a fork. Stir in the onion, garlic, and cilantro, if using.
- ❖ Serve with slices of jicama to dip in guacamole.
- ❖ To store, place plastic wrap over the bowl of guacamole and refrigerate. The guacamole will keep for about 2 days.

142) CURRIED TOFU "EGG SALAD" PITAS

Preparation Time: 15 minutes   **Cooking Time:** 0 minutes   **Servings: 4**

Ingredients:
Sandwiches Ingredients:
- ✓ 1 pound extra-firm tofu, drained and patted dry
- ✓ 1/2 cup vegan mayonnaise, homemade or store-bought
- ✓ 1/4 cup chopped mango chutney, homemade or store-bought
- ✓ 2 teaspoons Dijon mustard
- ✓ 1 tablespoon hot or mild curry powder
- ✓ 1 teaspoon salt

Ingredients:
- ✓ 1/8 teaspoon ground cayenne
- ✓ ¾ cup shredded carrots
- ✓ 2 celery ribs, minced
- ✓ 1/4 cup minced red onion
- ✓ 8 small Boston or other soft lettuce leaves
- ✓ 4 (7-inchwhole wheat pita breads, halved

Directions:
- ❖ Crumble the tofu and place it in a large bowl.
- ❖ Add the mayonnaise, chutney, mustard, curry powder, salt, and cayenne
- ❖ Stir well until thoroughly mixed.
- ❖ Then carrots, celery, and onion and stir to combine
- ❖ Refrigerate for 30 minutes to allow the flavors to blend
- ❖ Tuck a lettuce leaf inside each pita pocket
- ❖ Spoon some tofu mixture on top of the lettuce, and serve.

143) GARDEN PATCH SANDWICHES ON MULTIGRAIN BREAD

Preparation Time: 15 minutes   **Cooking Time:** 0 minutes   **Servings: 4**

Ingredients:
- ✓ 1 pound extra-firm tofu, drained and patted dry
- ✓ 1 medium red bell pepper, finely chopped
- ✓ 1 celery rib, finely chopped
- ✓ 3 green onions, minced
- ✓ 1/4 cup shelled sunflower seeds
- ✓ 1/2 cup vegan mayonnaise, homemade or store-bought

Ingredients:
- ✓ 1/2 teaspoon salt
- ✓ 1/2 teaspoon celery salt
- ✓ 1/4 teaspoon freshly ground black pepper
- ✓ 8 slices whole grain bread
- ✓ 4 (1/4-inchslices ripe tomato
- ✓ 4 lettuce leaves

Directions:
- ❖ Crumble the tofu and place it in a large bowl
- ❖ Add the bell pepper, celery, green onions, and sunflower seeds
- ❖ Stir in the mayonnaise, salt, celery salt, and pepper and mix until well combined.
- ❖ Toast the bread, if desired. Spread the mixture evenly onto 4 slices of the bread
- ❖ Top each with a tomato slice, lettuce leaf, and the remaining bread
- ❖ Cut the sandwiches diagonally in half and serve.

144) GARDEN SALAD WRAPS

Preparation Time: 15 minutes   **Cooking Time:** 10 minutes   **Servings: 4wraps**

Ingredients:
- ✓ 6 tablespoons olive oil
- ✓ 1 pound extra-firm tofu, drained, patted dry, and cut into 1⁄2-inch strips
- ✓ 1 tablespoon soy sauce
- ✓ 1⁄4 cup apple cider vinegar
- ✓ 1 teaspoon yellow or spicy brown mustard
- ✓ 1⁄2 teaspoon salt
- ✓ 1⁄4 teaspoon freshly ground black pepper

Directions:
- ❖ In a large skillet, heat 2 tablespoons of the oil over medium heat
- ❖ Add the tofu and cook until golden brown, about 10 minutes
- ❖ Sprinkle with soy sauce and set aside to cool.
- ❖ In a small bowl, combine the vinegar, mustard, salt, and pepper with the remaining 4 tablespoons oil
- ❖ Stir to blend well. Set aside.

Ingredients:
- ✓ 3 cups shredded romaine lettuce
- ✓ 3 ripe Roma tomatoes, finely chopped
- ✓ 1 large carrot, shredded
- ✓ 1 medium English cucumber, peeled and chopped
- ✓ 1⁄3 cup minced red onion
- ✓ 1⁄4 cup sliced pitted green olives
- ✓ 4 (10-inchwhole-grain flour tortillas or lavash flatbread

- ❖ In a large bowl, combine the lettuce, tomatoes, carrot, cucumber, onion, and olives
- ❖ Pour on the dressing and toss to coat.
- ❖ To assemble wraps, place 1 tortilla on a work surface
- ❖ Spread with about one-quarter of the salad
- ❖ Place a few strips of tofu on the tortilla and roll up tightly. Slice in half

145) TAMARI TOASTED ALMONDS

Preparation Time: 2 minutes   **Cooking Time:** 8 minutes   **Servings: ½ cup**

Ingredients:
- ✓ ½ cup raw almonds, or sunflower seeds
- ✓ 2 tablespoons tamari, or soy sauce

Ingredients:
- ✓ 1 teaspoon toasted sesame oil

Directions:
- ❖ Heat a dry skillet to medium-high heat
- ❖ Then add the almonds, stirring very frequently to keep them from burning
- ❖ Once the almonds are toasted, 7 to 8 minutes for almonds, or 3 to 4 minutes for sunflower seeds

- ❖ Pour the tamari and sesame oil into the hot skillet and stir to coat.
- ❖ You can turn off the heat, and as the almonds cool the tamari mixture will stick to and dry on the nuts.

146) TEMPEH-PIMIENTO CHEEZE BALL

Preparation Time: 5 minutes   **Cooking Time:** 30 minutes   **Servings: 8**

Ingredients:
- ✓ 8 ounces tempeh, cut into 1/2-inch pieces
- ✓ 1 (2-ouncejar chopped pimientos, drained
- ✓ 1/4 cup nutritional yeast

Ingredients:
- ✓ 1/4 cup vegan mayonnaise, homemade or store-bought
- ✓ 2 tablespoons soy sauce
- ✓ ¾ cup chopped pecans

Directions:
- ❖ In a medium saucepan of simmering water, cook the tempeh for 30 minutes
- ❖ Set aside to cool. In a food processor
- ❖ Combine the cooled tempeh, pimientos, nutritional yeast, mayo, and soy sauce
- ❖ Process until smooth.
- ❖ Transfer the tempeh mixture to a bowl and refrigerate until firm and chilled, at least 2 hours or overnight.
- ❖ In a dry skillet, toast the pecans over medium heat until lightly toasted, about 5 minutes. Set aside to cool.

- ❖ Shape the tempeh mixture into a ball, and roll it in the pecans
- ❖ Press the nuts slightly into the tempeh mixture so they stick
- ❖ Refrigerate for at least 1 hour before serving
- ❖ If not using right away, cover and keep refrigerated until needed
- ❖ Properly stored, it will keep for 2 to 3 days.

147) SAVORY ROASTED CHICKPEAS

Preparation Time: 5 minutes   **Cooking Time:** 25 minutes   **Servings: 1cup**

Ingredients:
- ✓ 1 (14-ouncecan chickpeas, rinsed and drained, or 1½ cups cooked
- ✓ 2 tablespoons tamari, or soy sauce
- ✓ 1 tablespoon nutritional yeast

Ingredients:
- ✓ 1 teaspoon smoked paprika, or regular paprika
- ✓ 1 teaspoon onion powder
- ✓ ½ teaspoon garlic powder

Directions:
- ❖ Preheat the oven to 400°F.
- ❖ Toss the chickpeas with all the other Ingredients, and spread them out on a baking sheet

- ❖ Bake for 20 to 25 minutes, tossing halfway through.
- ❖ Bake these at a lower temperature, until fully dried and crispy, if you want to keep them longer.

148) SAVORY SEED CRACKERS

Preparation Time: 5 minutes   **Cooking Time:** 50 minutes   **Servings: 20 crackers**

Ingredients:
- ✓ ¾ cup pumpkin seeds (pepitas
- ✓ ½ cup sunflower seeds
- ✓ ½ cup sesame seeds
- ✓ ¼ cup chia seeds
- ✓ 1 teaspoon minced garlic (about 1 clove)

Ingredients:
- ✓ 1 teaspoon tamari or soy sauce
- ✓ 1 teaspoon vegan Worcestershire sauce
- ✓ ½ teaspoon ground cayenne pepper
- ✓ ½ teaspoon dried oregano
- ✓ ½ cup water

Directions:
- ❖ Preheat the oven to 325°F.
- ❖ Line a rimmed baking sheet with parchment paper.
- ❖ In a large bowl, combine the pumpkin seeds, sunflower seeds, sesame seeds
- ❖ Then chia seeds, garlic, tamari, Worcestershire sauce, cayenne, oregano, and water.
- ❖ Transfer to the prepared baking sheet, spreading out to all sides.

- ❖ Bake for 25 minutes. Remove the pan from the oven
- ❖ Flip the seed "dough" over so the wet side is up
- ❖ Bake for another 20 to 25 minutes, until the sides are browned.
- ❖ Cool completely before breaking up into 20 pieces
- ❖ Divide evenly among 4 glass jars and close tightly with lids.

149) OMATO AND BASIL BRUSCHETTA

Preparation Time: 10 minutes   **Cooking Time:** 6 minutes   **Servings: 12 bruschetta**

Ingredients:
- ✓ 3 tomatoes, chopped
- ✓ ¼ cup chopped fresh basil
- ✓ 1 tablespoon olive oil

Ingredients:
- ✓ Pinch of sea salt
- ✓ 1 baguette, cut into 12 slices
- ✓ 1 garlic clove, sliced in half

Directions:
- ❖ In a small bowl, combine the tomatoes, basil, olive oil, and salt and stir to mix
- ❖ Set aside. Preheat the oven to 425°F.
- ❖ Place the baguette slices in a single layer on a baking
- ❖ Sheet and toast in the oven until brown, about 6 minutes.

- ❖ Flip the bread slices over once during cooking
- ❖ Remove from the oven and rub the bread on both sides with the sliced clove of garlic.
- ❖ Top with the tomato-basil mixture and serve immediately.

150) REFRIED BEAN AND SALSA QUESADILLAS

Preparation Time: 5 minutes   **Cooking Time:** 6 minutes   **Servings: 4 quesadillas**

Ingredients:
- ✓ 1 tablespoon canola oil, plus more for frying
- ✓ 11⁄2 cups cooked or 1 (15.5-ouncecan pinto beans, drained and mashed)
- ✓ 1 teaspoon chili powder

Ingredients:
- ✓ 4 (10-inchwhole-wheat flour tortillas
- ✓ 1 cup tomato salsa, homemade or store-bought
- ✓ 1/2 cup minced red onion (optional)

Directions:
- ❖ In a medium saucepan, heat the oil over medium heat.
- ❖ Add the mashed beans and chili powder
- ❖ Cook, stirring, until hot, about 5 minutes. Set aside.
- ❖ To assemble, place 1 tortilla on a work surface and spoon about 1/4 cup of the beans across the bottom half
- ❖ Top the beans with the salsa and onion, if using
- ❖ Fold top half of the tortilla over the filling and press slightly.

- ❖ In large skillet heat a thin layer of oil over medium heat.
- ❖ Place folded quesadillas, 1 or 2 at a time, into the hot skillet
- ❖ Heat until hot, turning once, about 1 minute per side.
- ❖ Cut quesadillas into 3 or 4 wedges and arrange on plates
- ❖ Serve immediately.

151) COCONUT CASHEW DIP

Preparation Time: 10 minutes   **Cooking Time:** 30 minutes   **Servings: 4**

Ingredients:
- ✓ ½ cup coconut cream
- ✓ 1 cup cashews, chopped
- ✓ 2 tablespoons cashew cheese, shredded

Ingredients:
- ✓ 1 teaspoon balsamic vinegar
- ✓ 1 tablespoon chives, chopped
- ✓ A pinch of salt and black pepper

Directions:
- ❖ In a pot, combine the cream with the cashew, cashew cheese and the other Ingredients

- ❖ Stir, cook over medium heat for 30 minutes and transfer to a blender.
- ❖ Pulse well, divide into bowls and serve.

152) SPICED OKRA BITES

Preparation Time: 10 minutes   **Cooking Time:** 15 minutes   **Servings: 4**

Ingredients:
- ✓ 2 cups okra, sliced
- ✓ 2 tablespoons avocado oil
- ✓ ¼ teaspoon chili powder
- ✓ ¼ teaspoon mustard powder

Ingredients:
- ✓ ¼ teaspoon garlic powder
- ✓ ¼ teaspoon onion powder
- ✓ A pinch of salt and black pepper

Directions:
- ❖ Spread the okra on a baking sheet lined with parchment paper
- ❖ Add the oil and the other Ingredients
- ❖ Toss and roast at 400 degrees F for 15 minutes.
- ❖ Divide the okra into bowls and serve as a snack.

153) ROSEMARY CHARD DIP

Preparation Time: 10 minutes   **Cooking Time:** 20 minutes   **Servings: 4**

Ingredients:
- ✓ 4 cups chard, chopped
- ✓ 2 cups coconut cream
- ✓ ½ cup cashews, chopped
- ✓ A pinch of salt and black pepper

Ingredients:
- ✓ 1 teaspoon smoked paprika
- ✓ ½ teaspoon chili powder
- ✓ ¼ teaspoon mustard powder
- ✓ ½ cup cilantro, chopped

Directions:
- ❖ In a pan, combine the chard with the cream, cashews and the other Ingredients
- ❖ Stir, cook over medium heat for 20 minutes and transfer to a blender.
- ❖ Pulse well, divide into bowls and serve as a party dip.

154) SPINACH AND CHARD HUMMUS

Preparation Time: 10 minutes   **Cooking Time:** 10 minutes   **Servings: 4**

Ingredients:
- ✓ 2 garlic cloves, minced
- ✓ 2 cup chard leaves
- ✓ 2 cups baby spinach
- ✓ ½ cup coconut cream

Ingredients:
- ✓ ¼ cup sesame paste
- ✓ A pinch of salt and black pepper
- ✓ 2 tablespoons olive oil
- ✓ Juice of ½ lemon

Directions:
- ❖ Put the cream in a pan, heat it up over medium heat
- ❖ Add the chard, garlic and the other Ingredients
- ❖ Stir, cook for 10 minutes, blend using an immersion blender
- ❖ Divide into bowls and serve.

155) VEGGIE SPREAD

Preparation Time: 10 minutes   **Cooking Time:** 20 minutes   **Servings: 4**

Ingredients:
- ✓ 2 tablespoons olive oil
- ✓ 1 cup shallots, chopped
- ✓ 2 garlic cloves, minced
- ✓ ½ cup eggplant, chopped
- ✓ ½ cup red bell pepper, chopped

Ingredients:
- ✓ ¼ cup tomatoes, cubed
- ✓ 2 tablespoons coconut cream
- ✓ ¼ cup veggie stock
- ✓ Salt and black pepper to the taste

Directions:
- ❖ Heat up a pan with the oil over medium heat, add the shallots and the garlic and sauté for 5 minutes.
- ❖ Add the eggplant, tomatoes and the other Ingredients, stir and cook for 15 minutes more.
- ❖ Blend the mix a bit with an immersion blender, divide into bowls and serve cold as a party spread.

156) MUSHROOM FALAFEL

Preparation Time: 10 minutes   **Cooking Time:** 12 minutes   **Servings: 6**

Ingredients:
- ✓ 1 cup mushrooms, chopped
- ✓ 1 bunch parsley leaves
- ✓ 4 scallions, hopped
- ✓ 5 garlic cloves, minced
- ✓ 1 teaspoon coriander, ground

Directions:
- ❖ In your food processor, combine the mushrooms with the parsley
- ❖ Add the other Ingredients except the flour and the oil and pulse well.
- ❖ Transfer the mix to a bowl, add the flour
- ❖ Stir well, shape medium balls out of this mix and flatten them a bit.

Ingredients:
- ✓ A pinch of salt and black pepper
- ✓ ¼ teaspoon baking soda
- ✓ 1 teaspoon lemon juice
- ✓ 3 tablespoons almond flour
- ✓ 2 tablespoons avocado oil

- ❖ Heat up a pan with the over medium-high heat
- ❖ Then the falafels, cook them for 6 minutes on each side
- ❖ Drain excess grease using paper towels
- ❖ Arrange them on a platter and serve as an appetizer.

157) THAI SNACK MIX

Preparation Time: 15 minutes   **Cooking Time:** 90 minutes   **Servings: 4**

Ingredients:
- ✓ 5 cups mixed nuts
- ✓ 1 cup chopped dried pineapple
- ✓ 1 cup pumpkin seed
- ✓ 1 teaspoon onion powder
- ✓ 1 teaspoon garlic powder
- ✓ 2 teaspoons paprika
- ✓ 1/2 teaspoon ground black pepper
- ✓ 1 teaspoon of sea salt

Directions:
- ❖ Switch on the slow cooker, add all the ingredients in it except for dried pineapple and red pepper flakes

Ingredients:
- ✓ 1/4 cup coconut sugar
- ✓ 1/2 teaspoon red chili powder
- ✓ 1 tablespoon red pepper flakes
- ✓ 1/2 tablespoon red curry powder
- ✓ 2 tablespoons soy sauce
- ✓ 2 tablespoons coconut oil

- ❖ Stir until combined and cook for 90 minutes at high heat setting, stirring every 30 minutes.
- ❖ When done, spread the nut mixture on a baking sheet lined with parchment paper and let it cool.

158) ZUCCHINI FRITTERS

Preparation Time: 10 minutes   **Cooking Time:** 6 minutes   **Servings: 12**

Ingredients:
- ✓ 1/2 cup quinoa flour
- ✓ 3 1/2 cups shredded zucchini
- ✓ 1/2 cup chopped scallions
- ✓ 1/3 teaspoon ground black pepper

Directions:
- ❖ Squeeze moisture from the zucchini by wrapping it in a cheesecloth
- ❖ Then transfer it to a bowl.
- ❖ Add remaining ingredients, except for oil
- ❖ Stir until combined and then shape the mixture into twelve patties.

Ingredients:
- ✓ 1 teaspoon salt
- ✓ 2 tablespoons coconut oil
- ✓ 2 flax eggs

- ❖ Take a skillet pan, place it over medium-high heat
- ❖ Then oil and when hot, add patties
- ❖ Cook for 3 minutes per side until brown.
- ❖ Serve the patties with favorite vegetarian sauce

159)   ZUCCHINI CHIPS

Preparation Time: 10 minutes   **Cooking Time:** 120 minutes   **Servings: 4**

Ingredients:
- ✓ 1 Large zucchini, thinly sliced
- ✓ 1 Teaspoon Salt

Ingredients:
- ✓ 2 Tablespoons olive oil

Directions:
- ❖ Pat dry zucchini slices and then spread them in an even layer on a baking sheet lined with parchment sheet.
- ❖ Whisk together salt and oil, brush this mixture over zucchini slices on both sides
- ❖ Bake for 2 hours or more until brown and crispy.

- ❖ When done, let the chips cool for 10 minutes
- ❖ Then serve straight away

160)   ROSEMARY BEET CHIPS

Preparation Time: 10 minutes   **Cooking Time:** 20 minutes   **Servings: 3**

Ingredients:
- ✓ 3 Large beets, scrubbed, thinly sliced
- ✓ 1/8 teaspoon ground black pepper
- ✓ ¼ teaspoon of sea salt

Ingredients:
- ✓ 3 sprigs of rosemary, leaves chopped
- ✓ 4 tablespoons olive oil

Directions:
- ❖ Spread beet slices in a single layer between two large baking sheets
- ❖ Brush the slices with oil, then season with spices and rosemary

- ❖ Toss until well coated, and bake for 20 minutes at 375 degrees F until crispy, turning halfway.
- ❖ When done, let the chips cool for 10 minutes and then serve.

DINNER RECIPES

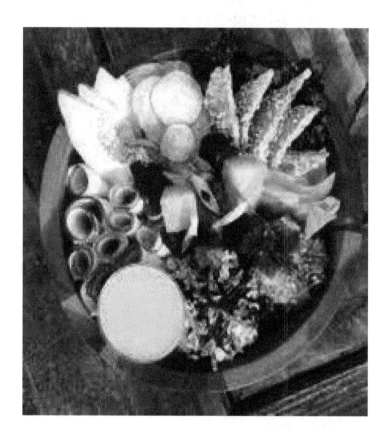

161)   SEITAN ZOODLE BOWL

Preparation Time: 15 minutes   **Cooking Time**: 13 minutes   **Servings: 4**

Ingredients:
- ✓ 5 garlic cloves, minced, divided
- ✓ ¼ tsp pureed onion
- ✓ Salt and ground black pepper to taste
- ✓ 2 ½ lb seitan, cut into strips
- ✓ 2 tbsp avocado oil
- ✓ 3 large eggs, lightly beaten

Ingredients:
- ✓ ¼ cup vegetable broth
- ✓ 2 tbsp coconut aminos
- ✓ 1 tbsp white vinegar
- ✓ ½ cup freshly chopped scallions
- ✓ 1 tsp red chili flakes
- ✓ 4 medium zucchinis, spiralized
- ✓ ½ cup toasted pine nuts, for topping

Directions:

- ❖ In a medium bowl, combine the half of the pureed garlic, onion, salt, and black pepper
- ❖ Add the seitan and mix well.
- ❖ Heat the avocado oil in a large, deep skillet over medium heat and add the seitan
- ❖ Cook for 8 minutes. Transfer to a plate.
- ❖ Pour the eggs into the pan and scramble for 1 minute
- ❖ Spoon the eggs to the side of the seitan and set aside.
- ❖ Reduce the heat to low and in a medium bowl
- ❖ Mix the vegetable broth, coconut aminos, vinegar, scallions

- ❖ Then remaining garlic, and red chili flakes.
- ❖ Mix well and simmer for 3 minutes.
- ❖ Stir in the seitan, zucchini, and eggs
- ❖ Cook for 1 minute and turn the heat off
- ❖ Adjust the taste with salt and black pepper.
- ❖ Spoon the zucchini food into serving plates
- ❖ Top with the pine nuts and serve warm.

162)   TOFU PARSNIP BAKE

Preparation Time: 5 minutes   **Cooking Time**: 44 minutes   **Servings: 4**

Ingredients:
- ✓ 6 vegan bacon slices, chopped
- ✓ 2 tbsp butter
- ✓ ½ lb parsnips, peeled and diced
- ✓ 2 tbsp olive oil
- ✓ 1 lb ground tofu
- ✓ Salt and ground black pepper to taste

Ingredients:
- ✓ 2 tbsp butter
- ✓ 1 cup full- fat heavy cream
- ✓ 2 oz dairy- free cream cheese (vegan), softened
- ✓ 1 ¼ cups grated cheddar cheese
- ✓ ¼ cup chopped scallions

Directions:

- ❖ Preheat the oven to 300 f and lightly grease a baking dish with cooking spray. Set aside.
- ❖ Put the vegan bacon in a medium pot and fry on both sides until brown and crispy, 7 minutes.
- ❖ Spoon onto a plate and set aside. Melt the butter in a large skillet
- ❖ Sauté the parsnips until softened and lightly browned
- ❖ Transfer to the baking sheet and set aside.
- ❖ Heat the olive oil in the same pan and cook the tofu
- ❖ (Seasoned with salt and black pepper)
- ❖ Spoon onto a plate and set aside too.

- ❖ Add the butter, full- fat heavy cream, cashew cream
- ❖ Then two-thirds of the cheddar cheese, salt, and black pepper to the pot
- ❖ Melt the ingredients over medium heat with frequent stirring, 7 minutes.
- ❖ Spread the parsnips in the baking dish, top with the tofu, pour the full- fat
- ❖ Heavy cream mixture over, and scatter the top with the vegan bacon and scallions.
- ❖ Sprinkle the remaining cheese on top
- ❖ Bake in the oven until the cheese melts and is golden, 30 minutes.
- ❖ Remove the dish, spoon the food into serving plates, and serve immediately

163) SQUASH TEMPEH LASAGNA

Preparation Time: 15 minutes   **Cooking Time:** 40 minutes   **Servings: 4**

Ingredients:
- ✓ 2 tbsp butter
- ✓ 1 ½ lb ground tempeh
- ✓ Salt and ground black pepper to taste
- ✓ 1 tsp garlic powder
- ✓ 1 tsp onion powder
- ✓ 2 tbsp coconut flour
- ✓ 1 ½ cup grated mozzarella cheese
- ✓ 1/3 cup parmesan cheese

Directions:
- ❖ Preheat the oven to 375 f and grease a baking dish with cooking spray. Set aside.
- ❖ Melt the butter in a large skillet over medium heat
- ❖ Cook the tempeh until brown, 10 minutes. Set aside to cool.
- ❖ In a medium bowl, mix the garlic powder, onion powder
- ❖ Add coconut flour, salt, black pepper
- ❖ Then mozzarella cheese, half of the parmesan cheese, cottage cheese, and egg. Set aside.
- ❖ In another bowl, combine the marinara sauce, mixed herbs
- ❖ Join also red chili flakes. Set aside.

Ingredients:
- ✓ 2 cups crumbled cottage cheese
- ✓ 1 large egg, beaten into a bowl
- ✓ 2 cups unsweetened marinara sauce
- ✓ 1 tbsp dried italian mixed herbs
- ✓ ¼ tsp red chili flakes
- ✓ 4 large yellow squash, sliced
- ✓ ¼ cup fresh basil leaves

- ❖ Make a single layer of the squash slices in the baking dish
- ❖ Spread a quarter of the egg mixture on top, a layer of the tempeh
- ❖ Then a quarter of the marinara sauce
- ❖ Repeat the layering process in the same ingredient proportions
- ❖ Sprinkle the top with the remaining parmesan cheese.
- ❖ Bake in the oven until golden brown on top, 30 minutes.
- ❖ Remove the dish from the oven, allow cooling for 5 minutes
- ❖ Garnish with the basil leaves, slice and serve.

164) BOK CHOY TOFU SKILLET

Preparation Time: 10 minutes   **Cooking Time:** 18 minutes   **Servings: 4**

Ingredients:
- ✓ 2 lb tofu, cut into 1-inch cubes
- ✓ Salt and ground black pepper to taste
- ✓ 4 vegan bacon slices, chopped
- ✓ 1 tbsp coconut oil

Directions:
- ❖ Season the tofu with salt and black pepper, and set aside.
- ❖ Heat a large skillet over medium heat and fry the vegan bacon until brown and crispy.
- ❖ Transfer to a plate.
- ❖ Melt the coconut oil in the skillet and cook the tofu
- ❖ (Until golden- brown and cooked through, 10 minutes
- ❖ Remove onto the vegan bacon plate and set aside.
- ❖ Add the bell pepper and bok choy to the skillet)

Ingredients:
- ✓ 1 orange bell pepper, deseeded, cut into chunks
- ✓ 2 cups baby bok choy
- ✓ 2 tbsp freshly chopped oregano
- ✓ 2 garlic cloves, pressed

- ❖ Sauté until softened, 5 minutes
- ❖ Stir in the vegan bacon, tofu, oregano, and garlic.
- ❖ Season with salt and black pepper
- ❖ Cook for 3 minutes or until the flavors incorporate.
- ❖ Turn the heat off.
- ❖ Plate the dish and serve with cauliflower rice.

165)   QUORN SAUSAGE FRITTATA

Preparation Time: 10 minutes   **Cooking Time:** 33 minutes   **Servings: 4**

Ingredients:
- ✓   12 whole eggs
- ✓   1 cup plain unsweetened yogurt
- ✓   Salt and ground black pepper to taste
- ✓   1 tbsp butter

Directions:
- ❖   Preheat the oven to 350 f.
- ❖   In a medium bowl, whisk the eggs, plain yogurt, salt, and black pepper.
- ❖   Melt the butter in a large (safe ovenskillet over medium heat)
- ❖   Sauté the celery until soft, 5 minutes. Transfer the celery into a plate and set aside.
- ❖   Add the quorn sausages to the skillet
- ❖   Cook until brown with frequent stirring to break the lumps that form, 8 minutes.

Ingredients:
- ✓   1 celery stalk, chopped
- ✓   12 oz quorn sausages
- ✓   ¼ cup shredded cheddar cheese

- ❖   Flatten the quorn sausage in the bottom of the skillet using the spoon
- ❖   Scatter the celery on top, pour the egg mixture all over
- ❖   Sprinkle with the cheddar cheese.
- ❖   Put the skillet in the oven
- ❖   Bake until the eggs set and cheese melts, 20 minutes.
- ❖   Remove the skillet, slice the frittata, and serve warm with kale salad.

166)   JAMAICAN JERK TEMPEH

Preparation Time: 15 minutes   **Cooking Time:** 45 minutes   **Servings: 4**

Ingredients:
- ✓   ½ cup plain unsweetened yogurt
- ✓   2 tbsp melted butter
- ✓   2 tbsp jamaican jerk seasoning salt and black pepper to taste

Directions:
- ❖   Preheat the oven to 350 f and grease a baking sheet with cooking spray.
- ❖   In a large bowl, combine the plain yogurt, butter, jamaican jerk seasoning, salt, and black pepper
- ❖   Add the tempeh and toss to coat evenly. Allow marinating for 15 minutes.
- ❖   In a food processor, blend the tofu with the almond meal until finely combined.
- ❖   Pour the mixture onto a wide plate.

Ingredients:
- ✓   2 lb tempeh
- ✓   3 tbsp tofu
- ✓   ¼ cup almond meal

- ❖   Remove the tempeh from the marinade, shake off any excess liquid
- ❖   Coat generously in the tofu mixture
- ❖   Place on the baking sheet and grease lightly with cooking spray.
- ❖   Bake in the oven for 40 to 45 minutes
- ❖   (Or until golden brown and crispy, turning once)
- ❖   Remove the tempeh and serve warm with red cabbage slaw and parsnip fries.

167) ZUCCHINI SEITAN STACKS

Preparation Time: 15 minutes   **Cooking Time**: 18 minutes   **Servings: 4**

Ingredients:
- ✓ 1 ½ lb seitan
- ✓ 3 tbsp almond flour
- ✓ Salt and black pepper to taste
- ✓ 2 large zucchinis, cut into

Directions:
- ❖ Preheat the oven to 400 f.
- ❖ Cut the seitan into strips and set aside.
- ❖ In a zipper bag, add the almond flour, salt, and black pepper
- ❖ Mix and add the seitan slices.
- ❖ Seal the bag and shake to coat the seitan with the seasoning.
- ❖ Grease a baking sheet with cooking spray
- ❖ Arrange the zucchinis on the baking sheet
- ❖ Season with salt and black pepper
- ❖ Drizzle with 2 tablespoons of olive oil.

Ingredients:
- ✓ 2-inch slices 4 tbsp olive oil
- ✓ 2 tsp italian mixed herb blend
- ✓ ½ cup vegetable broth

- ❖ Using tongs, remove the seitan from the almond flour mixture
- ❖ Shake off the excess flour, and put two to three seitan strips on each zucchini.
- ❖ Season with the herb blend and drizzle again with olive oil.
- ❖ Cook in the oven for 8 minutes
- ❖ Remove the sheet and carefully pour in the vegetable broth
- ❖ Bake further for 5 to 10 minutes or until the seitan cooks through.
- ❖ Remove from the oven and serve warm with low carb bread

168) CURRIED TOFU MEATBALLS

Preparation Time: 5 minutes   **Cooking Time**: 25 minutes   **Servings: 4**

Ingredients:
- ✓ 3 lb ground tofu
- ✓ 1 medium yellow onion, finely chopped
- ✓ 2 green bell peppers, deseeded and chopped
- ✓ 3 garlic cloves, minced
- ✓ 2 tbsp melted butter 1 tsp dried parsley

Directions:
- ❖ Preheat the oven to 400 f and grease a baking sheet with cooking spray.
- ❖ In a bowl, combine the tofu, onion, bell peppers, garlic, butter
- ❖ Add parsley, hot sauce, salt, black pepper, and curry powder.
- ❖ With your hands, form 1-inch tofu ball from the mixture
- ❖ Place on the greased baking sheet.

Ingredients:
- ✓ 2 tbsp hot sauce
- ✓ Salt and ground black pepper to taste
- ✓ 1 tbsp red curry powder
- ✓ 3 tbsp olive oil

- ❖ Drizzle the olive oil over the meat and bake in the oven
- ❖ (Until the tofu ball brown on the outside and cook within, 20 to 25 minutes)
- ❖ Remove the dish from the oven and plate the tofu ball.
- ❖ Garnish with some scallions
- ❖ Serve warm on a bed of spinach salad with herbed vegan paneer cheese dressing.

169)   SPICY MUSHROOM COLLARD WRAPS

Preparation Time: 10 minutes   **Cooking Time:** 16 minutes   **Servings: 4**

Ingredients:
- ✓ 2 tbsp avocado oil
- ✓ 1 large yellow onion, chopped
- ✓ 2 garlic cloves, minced
- ✓ Salt and ground black pepper to taste
- ✓ 1 small jalapeño pepper, deseeded and finely chopped

Directions:
- ❖ Heat 2 tablespoons of avocado oil in a large deep skillet
- ❖ Add and sauté the onion until softened, 3 minutes.
- ❖ Pour in the garlic, salt, black pepper, and jalapeño pepper
- ❖ Cook until fragrant, 1 minute.
- ❖ Mix in the mushrooms and cook both sides, 10 minutes.
- ❖ Add the cauliflower rice, and hot sauce

Ingredients:
- ✓ 1 ½ lb mushrooms, cut into 1-inch cubes
- ✓ 1 cup cauliflower rice
- ✓ 2 tsp hot sauce
- ✓ 8 collard leaves
- ✓ ¼ cup plain unsweetened yogurt for topping

- ❖ Sauté until the cauliflower slightly softens, 2 to 3 minutes
- ❖ Adjust the taste with salt and black pepper.
- ❖ Lay out the collards on a clean flat surface
- ❖ Spoon the curried mixture onto the middle part of the leaves, about 3 tablespoons per leaf
- ❖ Spoon the plain yogurt on top, wrap the leaves, and serve immediately.

170)   PESTO TOFU ZOODLES

Preparation Time: 5minutes   **Cooking Time:** 12minutes   **Servings: 4**

Ingredients:
- ✓ 2 tbsp olive oil
- ✓ 1 medium white onion, chopped
- ✓ 1 garlic clove, minced
- ✓ 2 (14 ozblocks firm tofu, pressed and cubed
- ✓ 1 medium red bell pepper, deseeded and sliced

Directions:
- ❖ Heat the olive oil in a medium pot over medium heat;
- ❖ Sauté the onion and garlic until softened and fragrant, 3 minutes.
- ❖ Add the tofu and cook until golden on all sides then pour in the bell pepper
- ❖ Cook until softened, 4 minutes.
- ❖ Mix in the zucchinis, pour the pesto on top

Ingredients:
- ✓ 6 medium zucchinis, spiralized
- ✓ Salt and black pepper to taste
- ✓ ¼ cup basil pesto, olive oil based
- ✓ 2/3 cup grated parmesan cheese
- ✓ ½ cup shredded mozzarella cheese toasted pine nuts to garnish

- ❖ Season with salt and black pepper
- ❖ Cook for 3 to 4 minutes or until the zucchinis soften a little bit
- ❖ Turn the heat off and carefully stir in the parmesan cheese.
- ❖ Dish into four plates, share the mozzarella cheese on top,
- ❖ Garnish with the pine nuts, and serve warm.

171)   CREAMY CAJUN ZUCCHINIS

Preparation Time: 10 minutes   **Cooking Time:** 20 minutes   **Servings: 4**

Ingredients:
- ✓ 1 pound zucchinis, roughly cubed
- ✓ 2 tablespoons olive oil
- ✓ 4 scallions, chopped
- ✓ Salt and black pepper to the taste

Directions:
- ❖ Heat up a pan with the oil over medium heat
- ❖ Add the scallions, cayenne and Cajun seasoning
- ❖ Stir and sauté for 5 minutes.

Ingredients:
- ✓ 1 teaspoon Cajun seasoning
- ✓ A pinch of cayenne pepper
- ✓ 1 cup coconut cream
- ✓ 1 tablespoon dill, chopped

- ❖ Then the zucchinis and the other Ingredients, toss
- ❖ Cook over medium heat for 15 minutes more
- ❖ Divide between plates and serve.

172) MASALA BRUSSELS SPROUTS

Preparation Time: 10 minutes   **Cooking Time:** 35 minutes   **Servings: 4**

Ingredients:
- ✓ 1 pound Brussels sprouts, trimmed and halved
- ✓ Salt and black pepper to the taste
- ✓ 1 tablespoon garam masala

Ingredients:
- ✓ 2 tablespoons olive oil
- ✓ 1 tablespoon caraway seeds

Directions:
- ❖ In a roasting pan, combine the sprouts with the masala
- ❖ Add the other ingredients, toss
- ❖ Bake at 400 degrees F for 35 minutes.
- ❖ Divide the mix between plates and serve.

173) NUTMEG GREEN BEANS

Preparation Time: 10 minutes   **Cooking Time:** 30 minutes   **Servings: 4**

Ingredients:
- ✓ 2 tablespoons olive oil
- ✓ ½ cup coconut cream
- ✓ 1 pound green beans, trimmed and halved
- ✓ 1 teaspoon nutmeg, ground

Ingredients:
- ✓ A pinch of salt and cayenne pepper
- ✓ ½ teaspoon onion powder
- ✓ ½ teaspoon garlic powder
- ✓ 2 tablespoons parsley, chopped

Directions:
- ❖ Heat up a pan with the oil over medium heat
- ❖ Add the green beans, nutmeg and the other ingredients, toss
- ❖ Cook for 30 minutes
- ❖ Divide the mix between plates and serve.

174) PEPPERS AND CELERY SAUTÉ

Preparation Time: 10 minutes   **Cooking Time:** 15 minutes   **Servings: 4**

Ingredients:
- ✓ 1 red bell pepper, cut into medium chunks
- ✓ 1 green bell pepper, cut into medium chunks
- ✓ 1 celery stalk, chopped
- ✓ 2 scallions, chopped
- ✓ 2 tablespoons olive oil

Ingredients:
- ✓ Salt and black pepper to the taste
- ✓ 1 tablespoons parsley, chopped
- ✓ 1 teaspoon cumin, ground
- ✓ 2 garlic cloves, minced

Directions:
- ❖ Heat up a pan with the oil over medium heat
- ❖ Add the scallions, garlic and cumin and sauté for 5 minutes.
- ❖ Then the peppers, celery and the other Ingredients, toss
- ❖ Cook over medium heat for 10 minutes more
- ❖ Divide between plates and serve.

175) CUCUMBER AND CAULIFLOWER MIX

Preparation Time: 10 minutes   **Cooking Time:** 12 minutes   **Servings: 4**

Ingredients:
- ✓ 1 cucumber, cubed
- ✓ 1 pound cauliflower florets
- ✓ 1 spring onion, chopped 2 tablespoons avocado oil
- ✓ 1 tablespoon balsamic vinegar

Ingredients:
- ✓ ¼ teaspoon red pepper flakes
- ✓ Salt and black pepper to the taste
- ✓ 1 tablespoon thyme, chopped

Directions:
- ❖ Heat up a pan with the oil over medium heat
- ❖ Add the spring onions and the pepper flakes and sauté for 2 minutes.
- ❖ Then the cucumber and the other ingredients, toss

- ❖ Cook over medium heat for 10 minutes more
- ❖ Divide between plates and serve.

176) GINGER MUSHROOMS

Preparation Time: 10 minutes   **Cooking Time:** 30 minutes   **Servings: 4**

Ingredients:
- ✓ 2 tablespoons coconut oil, melted
- ✓ 1 pound baby mushrooms
- ✓ Salt and black pepper to the taste

Ingredients:
- ✓ 1 tablespoon chives, chopped
- ✓ 2 tablespoons ginger, grated
- ✓ 1 teaspoon garlic powder

Directions:
- ❖ In a roasting pan, combine the mushrooms with the oil
- ❖ Add the other ingredients, toss

- ❖ Bake at 390 degrees F for 30 minutes.
- ❖ Divide the mix between plates and serve.

177) ENDIVE SAUTÉ

Preparation Time: 5 minutes   **Cooking Time:** 15 minutes   **Servings: 4**

Ingredients:
- ✓ 3 endives, shredded
- ✓ 1 tablespoon olive oil
- ✓ 4 scallions, chopped
- ✓ ½ cup tomato sauce

Ingredients:
- ✓ 2 garlic cloves, minced
- ✓ A pinch of sea salt and black pepper
- ✓ 1/8 teaspoon turmeric powder
- ✓ 1 tablespoon chives, chopped

Directions:
- ❖ Heat up a pan with the oil over medium heat
- ❖ Add the scallions and the garlic and sauté for 5 minutes.
- ❖ Then the endives and the other ingredients, toss

- ❖ Cook everything for 10 minutes more
- ❖ Divide between plates and serve.

178) ZUCCHINI PAN

Preparation Time: 5 minutes   **Cooking Time:** 20 minutes   **Servings: 4**

Ingredients:
- ✓ 1 pound zucchinis, sliced 1 yellow onion, chopped 2 tablespoons olive oil
- ✓ 2 apples, peeled, cored and cubed 1 tomato, cubed

Ingredients:
- ✓ 1 tablespoon rosemary, chopped 1 tablespoon chives, chopped

Directions:
- ❖ Heat up a pan with the oil over medium heat
- ❖ Add the onion and sauté for 5 minutes.

- ❖ Then the zucchinis and the other Ingredients, toss
- ❖ Cook over medium heat for 15 minutes more
- ❖ Divide between plates and serve.

179) GINGER MUSHROOMS

Preparation Time: 10 minutes   **Cooking Time:** 20 minutes   **Servings: 4**

Ingredients:
- ✓ 1 pound mushrooms, sliced
- ✓ 1 yellow onion, chopped
- ✓ 1 tablespoon ginger, grated
- ✓ 1 tablespoon olive oil
- ✓ 2 tablespoons balsamic vinegar

Ingredients:
- ✓ 2 garlic cloves, minced
- ✓ A pinch of salt and black pepper
- ✓ ¼ cup lime juice
- ✓ 2 tablespoons walnuts, chopped

Directions:
- ❖ Heat up a pan with the oil over medium-high heat
- ❖ Add the onion and the ginger and sauté for 5 minutes.
- ❖ Then the mushrooms and the other ingredients, toss
- ❖ Cook over medium heat for 15 minutes more
- ❖ Divide between plates and serve.

180) BELL PEPPER SAUTÉ

Preparation Time: 5 minutes   **Cooking Time:** 20 minutes   **Servings: 4**

Ingredients:
- ✓ 1 red bell pepper, cut into strips
- ✓ 1 yellow bell pepper, cut into strips
- ✓ 1 green bell pepper, cut into strips
- ✓ 1 orange bell pepper, cut into strips
- ✓ 3 scallions, chopped

Ingredients:
- ✓ 1 tablespoon olive oil
- ✓ 1 tablespoon coconut aminos
- ✓ A pinch of salt and black pepper
- ✓ 1 tablespoon parsley, chopped
- ✓ 1 tablespoon rosemary, chopped

Directions:
- ❖ Heat up a pan with the oil over medium-high heat
- ❖ Add the scallions and sauté for 5 minutes.
- ❖ Then the bell peppers and the other Ingredients, toss
- ❖ Cook over medium heat for 15 minutes more
- ❖ Divide between plates and serve.

DESSERT RECIPES

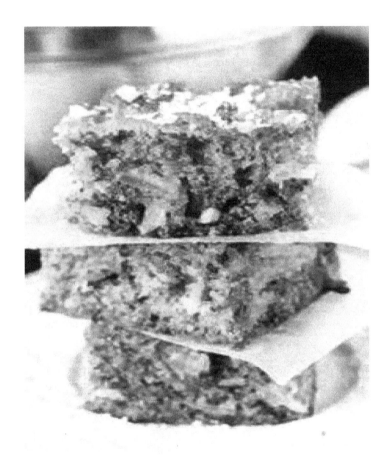

181) WARM RUM BUTTER SPICED CIDER

Preparation Time: 15 Minutes   **Cooking Time:** As per directions   **Servings: 4**

Ingredients:
- ✓ 3/4 cup rum
- ✓ 4 cups apple cider
- ✓ 2 cinnamon sticks
- ✓ 4 cardamom pods

Directions:
- ❖ Combine all the Ingredients in the instant pot

Ingredients:
- ✓ 1/4 teaspoon ground allspice
- ✓ 4 whole cloves
- ✓ 1 teaspoon lime juice
- ✓ 4 teaspoons nondairy butter

- ❖ Seal the lid and cook on high 5 minutes
- ❖ Let the pressure release naturally.

182) PEPPERMINT PATTY COCOA

Preparation Time: 15 Minutes   **Cooking Time:** As per directions   **Servings: 4**

Ingredients:
- ✓ 4 cups almond milk
- ✓ 3 ounces semisweet chocolate chips
- ✓ 1 teaspoon cocoa powder
- ✓ 1 teaspoon vanilla extract

Directions:
- ❖ Combine all the Ingredients in the instant pot
- ❖ Seal the lid and cook on high 4 minutes

Ingredients:
- ✓ 1/4 cup sugar
- ✓ 1 tablespoon agave nectar
- ✓ 1 teaspoon peppermint extract

- ❖ Then let the pressure release naturally.
- ❖ Serve garnished with a sprig of mint or topped with vegan marshmallows!

183) APPLE & WALNUT CAKE

Preparation Time: 20 Minutes   **Cooking Time:** As per directions   **Servings: 6**

Ingredients:
- ✓ 1¾ cups unbleached all-purpose flour
- ✓ 1 cup unsweetened applesauce
- ✓ ⅔ cup packed light brown sugar
- ✓ ½ cup chopped walnuts
- ✓ ¼ cup vegetable oil
- ✓ 1 tablespoon freshly squeezed lemon juice
- ✓ 1 teaspoon pure vanilla extract

Directions:
- ❖ Lightly oil a baking tray that will fit in the steamer basket of your Instant Pot.
- ❖ In a bowl, combine the flour, baking powder, baking soda
- ❖ Add sugar, cinnamon, allspice, nutmeg, cloves, and salt.
- ❖ In another bowl combine the applesauce, oil, vanilla, and lemon juice.
- ❖ Stir the wet mixture into the dry mixture slowly until they form a smooth mix.

Ingredients:
- ✓ 1½ teaspoons ground cinnamon
- ✓ 1 teaspoon baking powder
- ✓ ½ teaspoon baking soda
- ✓ ½ teaspoon salt
- ✓ ¼ teaspoon ground allspice
- ✓ ¼ teaspoon ground nutmeg
- ✓ ⅛ teaspoon ground cloves

- ❖ Fold in the walnuts.
- ❖ Pour the batter into your baking tray and put the tray in your steamer basket.
- ❖ Pour the minimum amount of water into the base of your Instant Pot and lower the steamer basket.
- ❖ Seal and cook on Steam for 12 minutes.
- ❖ Release the pressure quickly and set to one side to cool a little.

184) FAT FREE APPLE CAKE

Preparation Time: 20 Minutes   **Cooking Time:** As per directions   **Servings: 8**

Ingredients:
- ✓ 2 granny smith apples, peeled, cored, and diced
- ✓ 1¾ cups unbleached all-purpose flour
- ✓ ⅔ cup packed light brown sugar
- ✓ ½ cup applesauce
- ✓ 1 tablespoon freshly squeezed lemon juice
- ✓ 1½ teaspoons ground cinnamon
- ✓ 1 teaspoon pure vanilla extract

Ingredients:
- ✓ 1 teaspoon baking powder
- ✓ ½ teaspoon baking soda
- ✓ ½ teaspoon salt
- ✓ ¼ teaspoon ground allspice
- ✓ ¼ teaspoon ground nutmeg
- ✓ ⅛ teaspoon ground cloves

Directions:
- ❖ Lightly oil a baking tray that will fit in the steamer basket of your Instant Pot.
- ❖ In a bowl, combine the flour, baking powder, baking soda
- ❖ Add sugar, cinnamon, allspice, nutmeg, cloves, and salt.
- ❖ In another bowl combine the applesauce, vanilla, and lemon juice.
- ❖ Fold in the diced apples.
- ❖ Stir the wet mixture into the dry mixture slowly until they form a smooth mix.
- ❖ Pour the batter into your baking tray and put the tray in your steamer basket.
- ❖ Pour the minimum amount of water into the base of your Instan
- ❖ Pot and lower the steamer basket.
- ❖ Seal and cook on Steam for 12 minutes.
- ❖ Release the pressure quickly and set to one side to cool a little.

185) PINA-COLADA CAKE

Preparation Time: 20 Minutes   **Cooking Time:** As per directions   **Servings: 6**

Ingredients:
- ✓ 2 cups unbleached all-purpose flour
- ✓ 1 cup cream of coconut
- ✓ 1 cup confectioners' sugar
- ✓ ¾ cup canned pineapple, well drained, juice reserved
- ✓ ⅓ cup packed light brown sugar or granulated natural sugar
- ✓ ¼ cup unsweetened shredded coconut

Ingredients:
- ✓ 3 tablespoons vegan butter, softened, or vegetable oil
- ✓ 1 tablespoon dark rum or 1 teaspoon rum extract
- ✓ 1½ teaspoons baking powder
- ✓ 1 teaspoon apple cider vinegar
- ✓ ½ teaspoon salt
- ✓ ½ teaspoon baking soda
- ✓ ½ teaspoon coconut extract

Directions:
- ❖ Lightly oil a baking tray that will fit in the steamer basket of your Instant Pot.
- ❖ In a bowl combine the flour, sugar, shredded coconut
- ❖ Then baking soda, baking powder, and salt.
- ❖ In another bowl combine the cream of coconut, pineapple
- ❖ Add juice and flesh, rum, vinegar, and coconut extract.
- ❖ Combine the wet and dry mixes
- ❖ Stir well to ensure they are evenly combined.
- ❖ Pour the batter into your baking tray
- ❖ Put the tray in your steamer basket.
- ❖ Pour the minimum amount of water into the base of your Instant Pot and lower the steamer basket.
- ❖ Seal and cook on Steam for 12 minutes.
- ❖ Release the pressure quickly and set to one side to cool a little.
- ❖ When the cake is cool glaze with a light mix of confectioners' sugar and water.

186)   PUMPKIN SPICE CAKE

Preparation Time: 28 Minutes   **Cooking Time:** As per directions   **Servings: 6**

Ingredients:
- ✓ 1¾ cups unbleached all-purpose flour
- ✓ 1 cup canned solid-pack pumpkin
- ✓ ¾ cup packed light brown sugar or granulated natural sugar
- ✓ ½ cup chopped pecans
- ✓ ¼ cup unsweetened almond milk
- ✓ ¼ cup vegetable oil
- ✓ 1½ teaspoons baking powder

Ingredients:
- ✓ 1 teaspoon ground cinnamon
- ✓ 1 teaspoon pure vanilla extract
- ✓ ½ teaspoon salt
- ✓ ½ teaspoon ground nutmeg
- ✓ ½ teaspoon ground allspice
- ✓ ¼ teaspoon ground cloves

Directions:
- ❖ Lightly oil a baking tray that will fit in the steamer basket of your Instant Pot.
- ❖ In a bowl combine the flour, baking powder, cinnamon
- ❖ Then nutmeg, allspice, cloves, sugar, and salt.
- ❖ In another bowl combine the pumpkin, oil, almond milk, and vanilla.
- ❖ Mix the wet and dry mixtures together until the mix is evenly smooth.
- ❖ Fold in the pecans.

- ❖ Pour the batter into your baking tray
- ❖ Put the tray in your steamer basket.
- ❖ Pour the minimum amount of water into the base of your Instant Pot and lower the steamer basket.
- ❖ Seal and cook on Steam for 12 minutes.
- ❖ Release the pressure quickly and set to one side to cool a little.

187)   FUDGY CHOCOLATE CAKE

Preparation Time: 20 Minutes   **Cooking Time:** As per directions   **Servings: 8**

Ingredients:
- ✓ Cake:
- ✓ 1½ cups unbleached all-purpose flour
- ✓ 1 cup non-dairy milk
- ✓ 2/3 cup granulated natural sugar
- ✓ ¼ cup unsweetened cocoa powder
- ✓ 3 tablespoons vegan butter, softened
- ✓ 1½ teaspoons baking powder
- ✓ 1 teaspoon pure vanilla extract
- ✓ ½ teaspoon cider vinegar

Ingredients:
- ✓ ¼ teaspoon salt
- ✓ ¼ teaspoon baking soda
- ✓ Frosting:
- ✓ 1½ cups confectioners' sugar, plus more if needed
- ✓ ¼ cup unsweetened cocoa powder
- ✓ 2 tablespoons vegan butter, melted
- ✓ 3 tablespoons non-dairy milk, plus more if needed
- ✓ 1 teaspoon pure vanilla extract

Directions:
- ❖ Lightly oil a baking tray that will fit in the steamer basket of your Instant Pot.
- ❖ In a bowl combine the flour, cocoa powder, baking soda, baking powder, and salt.
- ❖ Whisk the vegan butter and granulated sugar until they form a creamy blend.
- ❖ Add the milk, vinegar, and vanilla.
- ❖ Then the flour mixture and stir until evenly mixed.
- ❖ Pour the batter into your baking tray and put the tray in your steamer basket.

- ❖ Pour the minimum amount of water into the base of your Instant Pot and lower the steamer basket.
- ❖ Seal and cook on Steam for 12 minutes.
- ❖ Release the pressure quickly and set to one side to cool a little.
- ❖ For the frosting, stir the cocoa into the melted butter until smoothly blended.
- ❖ Add the milk and vanilla and mix well again.
- ❖ Stir in the sugar until you have an almost pourable frosting.
- ❖ Refrigerate until it's time to frost your cake.

188)   CARROT & PINEAPPLE CAKE

Preparation Time: 20 Minutes   **Cooking Time:** As per directions   **Servings: 6**

Ingredients:
- ✓ 1½ cups unbleached all-purpose flour
- ✓ 2 carrots, peeled and finely shredded (1 cup packed
- ✓ ¾ cup packed light brown sugar or granulated natural sugar
- ✓ ½ cup pineapple juice from the chopped pineapple
- ✓ ½ cup chopped macadamia nuts
- ✓ ⅓ cup canned pineapple, well drained, juice reserved

Ingredients:
- ✓ ¼ cup vegetable oil
- ✓ 1½ teaspoons baking powder
- ✓ 1 teaspoon ground cinnamon
- ✓ ½ teaspoon salt
- ✓ ¼ teaspoon ground nutmeg

Directions:
- ❖ Lightly oil a baking tray that will fit in the steamer basket of your Instant Pot.
- ❖ In a bowl combine the flour, sugar, baking powder, cinnamon, nutmeg, and salt.
- ❖ In another bowl combine the carrot, pineapple, pineapple juice, and oil.
- ❖ Combine the wet and dry mix until a batter forms.
- ❖ Fold in the macadamias.
- ❖ Pour the batter into your baking tray and put the tray in your steamer basket.
- ❖ Pour the minimum amount of water into the base of your Instant Pot and lower the steamer basket.
- ❖ Seal and cook on Steam for 12 minutes.
- ❖ Release the pressure quickly and set to one side to cool a little.

189)   CREAM CHEESE FROSTING

Preparation Time: 5 Minutes   **Cooking Time:**   **Servings: 2.5 cups**

Ingredients:
- ✓ 1½ cups confectioners' sugar
- ✓ 1 cup vegan cream cheese at room temperature

Ingredients:
- ✓ ½ cup vegan butter, at room temperature
- ✓ 1 teaspoon pure vanilla extract

Directions:
- ❖ Combine all the Ingredients until smoothly blended.

190)   ORANGE POLENTA CAKE

Preparation Time: 30 Minutes   **Cooking Time:**   **Servings: 6**

Ingredients:
- ✓ 1¼ cups all-purpose flour
- ✓ 1 cup unsweetened almond milk
- ✓ 2/3 cup plus 1 tablespoon natural sugar
- ✓ ⅓ cup fine-ground cornmeal
- ✓ ⅓ cup plus 2 tablespoons marmalade
- ✓ ¼ cup finely ground almonds

Ingredients:
- ✓ ¼ cup vegan butter, softened
- ✓ 1 navel orange, peeled and sliced into ⅛-inch-thick rounds
- ✓ 1½ teaspoons baking powder
- ✓ 1 teaspoon pure vanilla extract
- ✓ ¾ teaspoon salt

Directions:
- ❖ Lightly oil a baking tray that will fit in the steamer basket of your Instant Pot.
- ❖ Sprinkle a tablespoon of sugar over the base of the baking tray and top with the orange slices.
- ❖ In a bowl combine the flour, cornmeal, baking powder, almonds, and salt.
- ❖ In another bowl combine the remaining sugar, the butter, 1/3 cup of marmalade
- ❖ Then vanilla and mix well. Slowly stir in the almond milk.
- ❖ Combine the wet and dry mixes into a smooth batter.
- ❖ Pour the batter into your baking tray and put the tray in your steamer basket.
- ❖ Pour the minimum amount of water into the base of your Instant Pot and lower the steamer basket.
- ❖ Seal and cook on Steam for 12 minutes.
- ❖ Release the pressure quickly and set to one side to cool a little.
- ❖ Warm the remaining 2 tablespoons of marmalade and brush over the cake.

191) SMOOTHIE BOWL

Preparation Time: 45 minutes   **Cooking Time:** As per directions   **Servings: 6**

Ingredients:
- ✓ 6 Oz. berries, fresh or frozen
- ✓ 2 medium frozen bananas
- ✓ ½ cup Almond milk
- ✓ 1 cup jellified yoghurt

Directions:
- ❖ In a blender mix the bananas with half of the berries until it has a puree consistency.

Ingredients:
- ✓ 1 tbsp. Chia seeds
- ✓ 1 tbsp. Hemp seeds
- ✓ 1 tbsp. Coconut flakes
- ✓ Raspberry jam or any other, to taste

- ❖ Organise your smoothie in a bowl decorating it in rows with the yogurt spot, the puree
- ❖ Then fresh berries and with a pinch of seeds and flakes you have.

192) COCONUT MILK SMOOTHIE

Preparation Time: 15 minutes   **Cooking Time:** As per directions   **Servings: 4**

Ingredients:
- ✓ 1 cup Greek yogurt
- ✓ 1 cup coconut milk, full fat
- ✓ 1 banana, fresh or frozen

Directions:
- ❖ In a blender mix all the ingredients until smooth

Ingredients:
- ✓ 1 cup baby spinach, fresh
- ✓ 1 tbsp. honey
- ✓ 5 Oz. blueberries or other berries

- ❖ Add the ice for a thicker smoothie.

193) YOGURT SMOOTHIE WITH CINNAMON AND MANGO

Preparation Time: 15 minutes   **Cooking Time:** As per directions   **Servings: 4**

Ingredients:
- ✓ 4 Oz. frozen mango chunks, mango pulp or fresh mango
- ✓ 1 cup Greek yogurt
- ✓ 1 cup coconut milk, full fat
- ✓ 3-4 cups milk

Directions:
- ❖ In a blender mix all the ingredients, except cinnamon until smooth

Ingredients:
- ✓ 3 tbsp. flax seed meal
- ✓ 1 tbsp. honey
- ✓ 1 tsp. cinnamon

- ❖ Sprinkle each smoothie with a pinch of cinnamon.

194) LEMON CURD DESSERT (SUGAR FREE)

Preparation Time: 35 minutes   **Cooking Time:** As per directions   **Servings: 4**

Ingredients:
- ✓ ½ cup unsalted butter
- ✓ ½ cup lemon juice
- ✓ 2 tbsp. lemon zest

Directions:
- ❖ 1On a low heat melt the butter in a saucepan.
- ❖ Whisk in the stevia or any other sweetener, lemon ingredients until combined
- ❖ Then add the egg yolks and return to the stove again over the low heat.

Ingredients:
- ✓ 6 egg yolks
- ✓ Stevia for sweetening

- ❖ Whisk it until the curd starts thickening.
- ❖ Strain into a small bowl and let cool.
- ❖ Can be stored in a fridge for several weeks.

195) CHOCOLATE ALMOND BUTTER SMOOTHIE

Preparation Time: 35 minutes   **Cooking Time:** As per directions   **Servings: 4**

Ingredients:
- ✓ 2 tbsp. chocolate protein powder
- ✓ ½ tbsp. cacao powder
- ✓ 1 cup almond milk
- ✓ 2 tbsp. almond butter

Directions:
- ❖ Put all the Ingredients into the blender

Ingredients:
- ✓ 1 fresh banana
- ✓ ½ cup fresh strawberries
- ✓ 1 tbsp. chia or hemp seeds
- ✓ Maple syrup or stevia for sweetening
- ❖ Mix until it has creamy consistency.

196) BERRY AND NUTS DESSERT

Preparation Time: 25 minutes   **Cooking Time:** As per directions   **Servings: 4**

Ingredients:
- ✓ 10 Oz. yogurt or yogurt drink
- ✓ 7 Oz. strawberries, fresh
- ✓ Blueberries, raspberries or any berries you may like
- ✓ 1 banana, sliced
- ✓ Pinch of Pistachio

Directions:
- ❖ In a serving dish pour the jellied yogurt

Ingredients:
- ✓ Pinch of cashews
- ✓ 4 walnuts, shelled
- ✓ Pinch of pumpkin seeds
- ✓ Pinch of sunflower seeds
- ✓ Several fresh mint leaves
- ❖ Top it with all the fresh ingredients

197) PASTRY WITH NUTS, MANGO AND BLUEBERRIES

Preparation Time: 45 minutes   **Cooking Time:** As per directions   **Servings: 6**

Ingredients:
For the pastry:
- ✓ 1 cup whole wheat flour
- ✓ ½ cup whole wheat almond flour
- ✓ ½ cup butter
- ✓ 2 eggs yolks
- ✓ 2 Oz. water
- ✓ 12 Oz. blueberries or any berries to your liking
- ✓ 2 Mangoes
- ✓ 1 pinch of pumpkin seeds

Ingredients:
- ✓ Sesame and sunflower seeds
- ✓ Peanuts, dried

For the filling:
- ✓ 8 Oz. cream cheese
- ✓ 1 mango, chopped
- ✓ ½ icing sugar
- ✓ 2 tbsp. lemon juice

Directions:
- ❖ In a bowl mix the flour ingredients with the butter
- ❖ Add the egg yolks and some water until combined and forms a ball.
- ❖ Knead the dough a little until it is smooth
- ❖ Refrigerate for half an hour covered with a napkin.
- ❖ Mix all the Ingredients of the pastry filling in a blender.

- ❖ Grease your baking tray or a cooking tin and dust with some flour.
- ❖ Pour the dough into the tin
- ❖ Bake for 30 minutes (200 grades) until lightly brown.
- ❖ Pour the filling onto the pastry and top it with berries and nuts
- ❖ Then some dessert sauce for serving.

198) VEGAN PUMPKIN MOUSSE

Preparation Time: 15 minutes   **Cooking Time:** As per directions   **Servings: 6**

Ingredients:
- ✓ 15 oz. firm Tofu
- ✓ 15 oz. organic Pumpkin
- ✓ 1 tbsp. Cinnamon

Ingredients:
- ✓ ½ tsp. Ginger
- ✓ Stevia for sweetening

Directions:
- ❖ Mix all the ingredients in a blender until smooth

- ❖ Taste and add more stevia for sweetening.

199) FLAX SEED WAFFLES

Preparation Time: 20 minutes   **Cooking Time:** As per directions   **Servings: 4**

Ingredients:
- ✓ 2 cups Golden Flax Seed
- ✓ 1 tbsp. Baking Powder
- ✓ 5 tbsp. Flax Seed Meal (mixed with 15 tbsp. Water)
- ✓ ⅓ cup Avocado Oil

Ingredients:
- ✓ ½ cup Water
- ✓ 1 tsp. Sea Salt
- ✓ 1 tbsp. fresh Herbs (thyme, rosemary or parsley) or 2 tsp. cinnamon, ground

Directions:
- ❖ Preheat the waffle-maker.
- ❖ Combine the flax seed with baking powder with a pinch of salt in a bowl
- ❖ Whisk the mixture.
- ❖ Place the jelly-like flax seed mixture, some water and oil into the blender and pulse until foamy.
- ❖ Transfer the liquid mixture to the bowl with the flax seed mixture
- ❖ Stir until combined. The mixture must be fluffy.
- ❖ Once it is combined, set aside for a couple of minutes

- ❖ Add some fresh herbs or cinnamon
- ❖ Divide the mixture into 4 servings.
- ❖ Scoop each, one at a time, onto the waffle maker
- ❖ Cook with the closed top until it's ready
- ❖ Repeat with the remaining batter.
- ❖ Eat immediately or keep in an air-tight container for a couple of weeks.

90

200) LEMON FAT BOMBS

Preparation Time: 60 minutes   **Cooking Time:** As per directions   **Servings: 4**

Ingredients:
- ✓ 1 cup Coconut Oil, melted
- ✓ 2 cups Raw Cashews, boiled for 10 minutes, soaked
- ✓ ½ cup Coconut Butter
- ✓ 1 Lemon Zest
- ✓ 2 Lemons, juiced

Directions:
- ❖ Mix all the Ingredients in a food processor and blend until combined.
- ❖ Place the mixture to a bowl and have it cooled up in the freezer to 40 minutes.
- ❖ Remove from freezer and make the balls.
- ❖ Place them onto the cooking tray and again

Ingredients:
- ✓ ¼ cup Coconut Flour
- ✓ ⅓ cup Coconut, shredded
- ✓ A pinch of salt
- ✓ Stevia for sweetening

- ❖ Put into the freezer for hardening.
- ❖ Remove from the freezer
- ❖ Store in an air-tight container for up to a week
- ❖ Let them thaw before serving.

Thanks for reading this book

CPSIA information can be obtained
at www.ICGtesting.com
Printed in the USA
BVHW011352210621
610125BV00009B/2507